An Appraisal of the Status of Chagas Disease in the United States

Rodrigo Zeledón

Charles B. Beard

J.C. Pinto Dias

David A. Leiby

Patricia L. Dorn

José Rodrigues Coura

ELSEVIER

AMSTERDAM • BOSTON • HEIDELBERG • LONDON
NEW YORK • OXFORD • PARIS • SAN DIEGO
SAN FRANCISCO • SINGAPORE • SYDNEY • TOKYO

Elsevier
Radarweg 29, Amsterdam, 1043 NX, Netherlands
225 Wyman Street, Waltham 02451, USA

First published 2012

Notices
Knowledge and best practice in this field are constantly changing. As new research and experience broaden our understanding, changes in research methods, professional practices, or medical treatment may become necessary.

Practitioners and researchers must always rely on their own experience and knowledge in evaluating and using any information, methods, compounds, or experiments described herein. In using such information or methods they should be mindful of their own safety and the safety of others, including parties for whom they have a professional responsibility.

To the fullest extent of the law, neither the publisher nor the authors, contributors, or editors assume any liability for any injury and/or damage to persons or property as a matter of products liability, negligence, or otherwise, or from any use or operation of any methods, products, instructions, or ideas contained in the material herein.

British Library Cataloguing-in-Publication Data
A catalogue record for this book is available from the British Library

Library of Congress Cataloging-in-Publication Data
A catalog record for this book is available from the Library of Congress

ISBN: 978-0-12-397268-2

For information on all Elsevier publications
visit our website at *elsevierdirect.com*

This book has been manufactured using Print On Demand technology. Each copy is produced to order and is limited to black ink. The online version of this book will show color figures where appropriate.

Printed and bound by CPI Group (UK) Ltd, Croydon, CR0 4YY

Transferred to Digital Print 2011

TABLE OF CONTENTS

DEDICATION

The authors are pleased to dedicate this monograph to three pioneer researchers whose work inspired others to undertake studies on many aspects of Chagas disease in the United States. First, to Professor Emmanuel Dias (deceased) from Brazil who, based on the epidemiological facts in 1951, suggested autochthonous vector transmission and identified chagasic cardiopathy in patients. Second, to Professors Sam F. Wood (deceased) and Raymond E. Ryckman, both from the United States, who in numerous publications, along with their respective groups, described much of the basic information important in the understanding of Chagas disease in the United States.

CHAPTER 1

Introduction and Historical Background

Chagas disease (American trypanosomiasis) was named after the Brazilian physician Carlos Justiniano Ribeiro Chagas, who in 1909 announced to the world the discovery of this new parasitic disease in animals and humans, in the town of Lassance, State of Minas Gerais, Brazil. In 1908, Chagas observed, for the first time, flagellate forms of the parasite in the intestine of the hematophagous bug *Panstrongylus megistus* (initially called *Conorhinus megistus*), which he found residing in human dwellings in Brazil. A few months later, he studied the parasite by experimentally infecting monkeys, rodents, and dogs. At the beginning of 1909, Chagas discovered the same flagellate in the blood of a cat and in a 2-year-old girl and realized that he had discovered a new disease-causing agent, transmitted by hemipteran insects in the family Reduviidae, subfamily Triatominae. He named the new trypanosome *Schizotrypanum cruzi*, which was later renamed *Trypanosoma cruzi*. The enzootic condition of the new trypanosomiasis was also demonstrated by Chagas after he found a natural infection in an armadillo (*Dasypus novemcinctus*) and a bug (*Panstrongylus geniculatus*) sharing the same burrow (Chagas, 1909a, 1909b, 1912; Coura, 1997).

According to the classical WHO data, it was estimated that Chagas disease affected 16–18 million people with at least 100 million at risk of contracting the infection in 21 countries throughout Latin America. There were an estimated 1 million new cases of chronic disease and some 45,000 deaths annually (WHO, 1991, 1995). Recent data indicate that these figures have been reduced drastically to less than 10 million, mainly due to the action of the various control "initiatives" throughout Latin America. Marked reductions in incidence and prevalence have been observed since the Southern Cone Initiative was launched in 1991, with consequent important savings in healthcare expenditures for the countries (Moncayo and Ortiz-Yanine, 2006; Schofield et al., 2006; Yamagata and Nakagawa, 2006). Likewise, the efforts toward the total elimination of *Rhodnius prolixus* from the Central American subregion, a target of the Central American Initiative, have been extremely successful (cf. Zeledón et al., 2008). In fact, the transmission of

An Appraisal of the Status of Chagas Disease in the United States. DOI: 10.1016/B978-0-12-397268-2.00001-8

Chagas disease by *R. prolixus* is presently considered to be interrupted in the entire subregion, due to its apparent elimination (OPS, 2011).

In the United States, the parasite was first observed in California in another species of bug, *Triatoma protracta*, a few years after Chagas' initial observation (Kofoid and McCulloch, 1916). Nevertheless, when these authors failed to find the blood forms in the natural host of the bug, the wood rat (*Neotoma fuscipes*), they thought that the flagellate they had found was a different species and named it *Trypanosoma triatomae*. Furthermore, according to Kofoid and Donat (1933a) at that time, they were unable to transmit the parasite to laboratory albino rats through the bite of the infected insects. Later on, Kofoid and Donat (1933a, 1933b) succeeded in infecting laboratory and wild *Neotoma* rats plus one opossum (*Didelphis virginiana*) through *T. protracta*-infected feces, demonstrating that the previously observed flagellate present in the bug was indeed the same trypanosome described by Chagas in Brazil several years earlier. These authors stressed the fact that, of the six subspecies of *N. fuscipes* present in California, they found that the bugs (*T. protracta*) in *Neotoma fuscipes macrotis* and *Neotoma fuscipes annectans* nests, but only those associated with the former wood rat were infected with *T. cruzi* (Kofoid and Donat, 1933b).

The experiments were extended by Wood (1934a, 1934b), who proved that in fact *Triatoma protracta* and *N. fuscipes* are natural hosts of the parasite, that it is possible to experimentally infect different mammals (including rhesus monkeys and dogs), that amastigotes are formed in tissues of the infected animals, and that the infections tend to be light, suggesting a low virulence of the trypanosome.

Also in the 1930s, *T. cruzi* infections were discovered in other species of bugs such as *Triatoma uhleri* (also known as *Triatoma rubida*) in Arizona (Kofoid and Whitaker, 1936) and *Triatoma sanguisuga* and *Triatoma gerstaeckeri* in Texas (Anonymous, 1938; Packchanian, 1939). Additional species were also later found infected as indicated below. An interesting antecedent is that *T. sanguisuga* was reported from the state of Georgia as early as 1855 by Le Conte, who made the observation that people, particularly children, were bitten by the bug there (Le Conte, 1855). The same species was confirmed in Georgia by Stal (1859) a few years later. Similarly, this species was found in beds and reported to bite humans in Illinois in counties such as Madison, Jersey, Union, and Adams (Walsh and Riley, 1869). Uhler (1876, 1878) made reference to *T. sanguisuga* as inhabiting Virginia, Maryland, Ohio, Texas, Florida, and Illinois and pointed out that it was a "blood-thirsty tenant of the beds in houses." Ryley and Howard (1892) presented evidence of *Conorhinus sanguisugus* (*T. sanguisuga*) biting humans in Missouri and Oklahoma (Indian Territory). In the latter place, the bugs were in a bed in a log house, and apparently representatives of the species were also reported in the forests. Kimball (1894) found this bug, in large numbers, in poultry houses and in barns attacking horses, and occasionally in houses in Manhattan, Kansas, causing serious allergic reactions in people. A similar situation was pointed out by Marlatt (1896) in parts of Texas and Kansas, where the insect was a frequent visitor of homes.

John Lembert made observations of humans bitten by *T. protracta* in the Yosemite Valley in the 1860s (Mortensen and Walsh, 1963). Thurman (1944) mentioned the first finding of *Triatoma neotomae* in Texas by Schwartz in 1898, even though the specimens were not properly identified at that time.

In 1899, there were several nationwide newspaper releases, originating with the story of a lady from Washington D.C. who developed a severe reaction when bitten on the face by one of these insects (*T. sanguisuga*). This seems to be the origin of the common name "kissing bug," used for the first time on that occasion (Howard, 1899; Shields and Walsh, 1956). Other common names found in the American literature are cone-nosed bug, bloodsucker, Mexican bed bug, China bug, and assassin bug.

Stal (1859) makes reference to other species of the same group being present in the United States, including *C. gerstaeckeri* and *C. variegatus* (aka *Triatoma lecticularia*) in Texas. Uhler (1876) also mentions the presence of the latter species in California, Georgia, Louisiana, and Illinois. Ryley and Howard (1893) reported that in Washington County, Florida, *T. lecticularia* "frequently fly into houses." Howard (1899) added that *C. protracta* was present in California, Arizona, and Utah and included Missouri in the distribution of *C. sanguisugus*.

Collectively, these reports demonstrate that triatomine vectors of Chagas diseases have existed in the United States, under wild conditions, for many centuries, and that some species have been associated with human dwellings for a long time, causing allergic reactions of varying degrees in people. Also, Barnabé et al. (2001), on the basis of phylogenetic studies, are of the opinion that *T. cruzi* not only is native to the

United States but also has been part of the native fauna for a very long time. Interestingly, Reinhard et al. (2003) suggest that a prehistoric mummy from the Chihuahuan Desert, at the Texas-Coahuila border, might represent an ancient North American case of Chagas disease. This individual presented intestinal alterations consistent with megacolon, a condition that can be associated with the disease.

Details on the distribution and infection of various bug species occurring in the United States are presented in this chapter along with the unique epidemiological aspects of Chagas disease in this region. Additionally, we present evidence that Chagas disease is a rather common zoonotic infection, involving many species of North American wild mammals, domestic pets, and, in a small but important number of instances, human beings. Even though we believe that human infection in the United States has been underestimated for years, the incidence and prevalence rates of the disease in the United States are clearly much lower than in endemic regions of Latin America, for reasons we will discuss.

CHAPTER 2

Triatomine Vectors

2.1 SPECIES AND DISTRIBUTION

The triatomine species in the United States are considered sylvatic, with most species living in association with rodent dens, particularly those of the genus *Neotoma*. Some species such as *T. sanguisuga* have also been found in tree bark or in palm trees, and for *Triatoma recurva* the habitat is unknown (see below). Following the binomial nomenclature of Lent and Wygodzinsky (1979), and disregarding the subspecies designations of other authors, there are 11 known species of triatomines reported as present in the United States, 10 belonging to the genus *Triatoma* and one to *Paratriatoma* (Table 2.1 and Figure 2.1, see Plate 1). One of these species, the cosmopolitan *Triatoma rubrofasciata*, was found only once in the continental United States, in Jacksonville, Florida, and is probably very uncommon (Usinger, 1944). Interestingly, this species has also been reported from Hawaii (Arnold and Bell, 1944) and is cited as present in the Virgin Islands (Ryckman, 1984). Another species, *Triatoma incrassata*, was only described from Arizona and also seems to be very rare (Ryckman, 1962). Of the 10 species found in the United States (excluding the cosmopolitan *T. rubrofasciata*), all are shared with Mexico, where, except *T. gerstaeckeri*, none of them has epidemiological importance (Cruz-Reyes and Pickering-López, 2006; Guzmán-Bracho, 2001; Martínez-Ibarra et al., 1992). Nevertheless, at present, *T. rubida* and *T. recurva* are becoming domestic and peridomestic species in the city of Guaymas, State of Sonora, in northwestern Mexico. Both species were found colonizing houses, and *T. rubida* was more common and showed high infection indexes for *T. cruzi* (Paredes et al., 2001; Pfeiler et al., 2006).

The presence of *T. sanguisuga* was doubtful for some time after being reported from the state of Mexico, but there are at least two reports of its existence in the states of Sinaloa and Chihuahua (Cruz-Reyes and Pickering-López, 2006; Ryckman and Casdin, 1976).

As can be observed in Table 2.1 and Figure 2.1 (see Plate 1), some species are more widely distributed than others. They have been found

An Appraisal of the Status of Chagas Disease in the United States. DOI: 10.1016/B978-0-12-397268-2.00002-X

Table 2.1. Species of Triatominae Bugs Found in the United States and Their Distribution by State

Species	Distribution	References
Paratriatoma hirsuta	Arizona, California, Colorado, Nevada, New Mexico	Ryckman, 1981; Wood, 1941a, 1941c
T. gerstaeckeri	New Mexico, Texas	Kjos et al., 2009; Packchanian, 1949; Wood and Wood, 1961
T. incrassata	Arizona	Ryckman, 1962
Triatoma indictiva	Arizona, New Mexico, Texas	Dias, 1951; Kjos et al., 2009; Lent and Wygodzinsky, 1979; Wood, 1941c
T. lecticularia (aka T. heidemanni)	Arizona, California, Florida, Georgia, Illinois, Kansas, Louisiana, Maryland, Missouri, New Mexico, North Carolina, Oklahoma, Pennsylvania, South Carolina, Tennessee, Texas	Carcavallo et al., 1999; Dias, 1951; Kjos et al., 2009; Packchanian, 1940a; Thurman et al., 1948; Wood, 1942a
T. neotomae	Texas	Kjos et al., 2009; Ryckman, 1986
T. protracta	Arizona, California, Colorado, Nevada, New Mexico, Texas, Utah	Ekkens, 1981; Klotz et al., 2009; Kjos et al., 2009; Reisenman et al., 2010; Usinger, 1939
T. recurva (aka T. longipes)	Arizona, California, Colorado, Nevada, New Mexico, Texas	Ikenga and Richerson, 1984; Ryckman, 1981, 1984; Wood, 1941a
T. rubida	Arizona, California, Colorado, Nevada, New Mexico, Texas	Dias, 1951; Ekkens, 1981; Kjos et al., 2009; Klotz et al., 2009; Reisenman et al., 2010; Ryckman, 1984; Wood, 1941a, 1941c, 1953a
T. rubrofasciata	Florida, Hawaii, Virgin Islands	Arnold and Bell, 1944; Ryckman, 1984; Usinger, 1939
T. sanguisuga	Alabama, Arizona, Arkansas, Florida, Georgia, Illinois, Indiana, Kansas, Kentucky, Louisiana, Maryland, Mississippi, Missouri, New Jersey, New Mexico, North Carolina, Ohio, Oklahoma, Pennsylvania, South Carolina, Tennessee, Texas, Virginia	Dias, 1951; Dorn et al., 2007; Kjos et al., 2009; Lent and Wygodzinsky, 1979; Nieto et al., 2009; Olsen et al., 1964; Porter, 1965; Readio, 1927; Ryckman and Casdin, 1976; Ryckman, 1984; Thurman et al., 1948; Usinger, 1944; Whittacker and Jarecka, 1974; Wood, 1942a

in 27 states throughout two-thirds of the United States. The most widely distributed species are *T. lecticularia*, present in 16 states and extending across the country from ocean to ocean, and *T. sanguisuga*, which occurs in 23 states, particularly those of the eastern half, as far north as Illinois, Indiana, Ohio, Pennsylvania, and New Jersey, all the way to Florida in the southeast and Arizona in the southwest but not reaching the Pacific coast. In Alabama alone, it has been found in at least 18 counties, and "the species may be found wherever suitable habitats occur" (Hays, 1966). Four species have been reported in five to seven states (*T. protracta*, *T. recurva*, *T. rubida*, and *P. hirsuta*); others are more restricted in their distribution. Arizona, New Mexico, and Texas are the states with the most

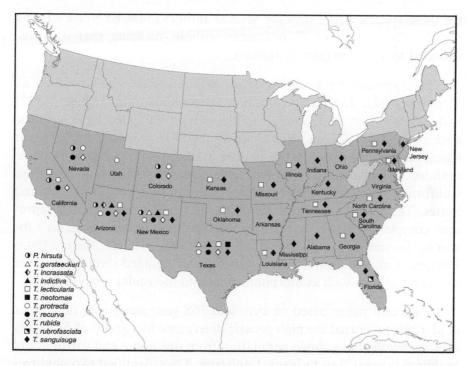

Figure 2.1. Geographic distribution of U.S. triatomine species. (See Plate 1).

species (eight each), followed by California with five and Nevada and Colorado with four. Ryckman (1984) believes that the reports of *T. sanguisuga* from Arizona and New Mexico more likely correspond to *T. indictiva* and that this species may extend northward to Ohio, West Virginia, and Kentucky; however, positive collection records "do not appear to be readily available."

Ryckman (1986) made an accurate assessment when he stated that the report of *T. neotomae* from Arizona, California, and New Mexico by Lent and Wygodzinsky (1979) "appear[s] to be in error." In fact, the mistake originated from confusion in the literature. Neiva (1911), in Brazil, described *T. uhleri* (aka *T. rubida*) and *T. neotomae* as new species. He mentioned Texas, Arizona, California, and New Mexico as the states where the first one was found, and Arizona and Texas as the states where the second was found, even though the three specimens he received for describing this species were all from Texas. In 1914, Neiva in his thesis reviewing the *Triatoma* genus attributed by mistake the distribution of *T. uhleri* to *T. neotomae*, mixing the previous notes for these species. From then on, several authors followed Neiva's thesis for the distribution of *T. neotomae* without realizing that it corresponded to *T. uhleri* (aka *T. rubida*).

The confusion by Uhler in 1876, between what was described as *T. longipes* (aka *T. recurva*) from San Diego, California (Usinger, 1939) and a dark variety of *Triatoma phyllosoma*, probably led some authors, such as Readio (1927) and Neiva and Lent (1941), to report this Mexican species as being present in the United States. Also, the report by later authors of *Dipetalogaster maxima*, a Mexican species indigenous to Baja California, should also be considered a mistaken record in the United States. The hypothesis that some of the North American species represent complexes of two or more species, previously considered as subspecies by some authors (Ryckman, 1962, 1967, 1971; Usinger, 1944; Usinger et al., 1966), will have to await more detailed studies based on the new methods such as morphometrics and molecular analysis.

In a recent paper based on cytb and 16S gene sequences, de la Rua et al. (2011) reported the high genetic divergence in a group of 54 adults of *T. sanguisuga* in a single population from one house and surrounding buildings in rural New Orleans, Louisiana. They identified two phylogenetic groups among the bugs, supporting the existence of a subspecies of *T. sanguisuga* corresponding to the first group. The authors discussed the importance of a "systematic study across its large geographic range," which "could clarify the taxonomic status of this species."

2.2 RELATIONSHIP WITH HUMAN DWELLINGS

The adaptation of certain species of triatomines to human dwellings is a slow and gradual process that likely depends on several entomologic, anthropocentric, and environmental factors (Forattini, 1980; Zeledón, 1974). In Central and South America, some species have been more successful than others, with the process being associated over several centuries with poor living conditions. The extreme is represented by *Triatoma infestans* and *R. prolixus* in South and Central America; these species are present in some areas exclusively in the domestic environment, where their populations reach high densities. Adaptations toward domesticity are in contrast to some rather uncommon species, mainly those belonging to the genera *Psammolestes* and *Cavernicola*, which are associated with birds, bats, or other small animals and rarely have contact with humans.

Other species found in the United States are in a middle category because they are essentially wild insects, with adults visiting human dwellings, and in some cases with a few nymphs found inside houses. There is some evidence in the literature to suggest that a few species are becoming better adapted to some of the loosely constructed or even standard dwellings with poor sanitary conditions and that perhaps the finding of colonies of the insects, either indoors or outdoors, may be an emerging condition in areas where the bugs have existed for many years (Barretto, 1979). Great numbers of triatomines (several hundreds or even thousands) colonizing in houses, as has occurred in disease-endemic areas of Central and South America (Dias and Zeledón, 1955; Sandoval et al., 2000), are not found in the United States. Nevertheless, as we will see later, the visitation of human dwellings, of different construction types, by flying adult insects, particularly in the warmer seasons, is not an uncommon phenomenon in certain regions of the country.

As already mentioned, there are some old reports indicating that a human–insect relationship has existed since the 19th century and even before, resulting over various annoyances associated with these bugs. The information accumulated over the past 60 years indicates that the problem is more common in some states than in others and that it deserves more careful attention in certain parts of the country. The present evidence suggests that colonies of insects might be more common in human dwellings than previously thought and may have been overlooked, at least in some localities.

In Table 2.2 and Figure 2.2 (see Plate 2), we summarize and illustrate the published data on the seven species that have been reported to frequently visit households in at least 12 states. Most of the reports make reference to adult insects that fly mainly at night, most commonly attracted to lights, entering homes or remaining in the peridomicile, sometimes in large numbers. Nevertheless, there are reports of at least six of these species (*T. gerstaeckeri*, *T. lecticularia*, *T. protracta*, *T. recurva*, *T. rubida*, and *T. sanguisuga*) collected as nymphs inside or very close to houses, indicating that they can colonize human dwellings (see Plate 3). This is an important epidemiological fact, suggesting that in some places where the sanitary condition of the houses are unsatisfactory the bugs may find the right conditions to thrive inside or in the periphery of the dwelling, creating the threat of increased risk of vectorial transmission of Chagas disease to people.

Table 2.2. Species of Triatomines Found in and Near Houses in the United States

Species	State	Location	Instars	References
P. hirsuta	California	Inside	Adults	Wood, 1942a
	Arizona	Inside	Adults	Wood, 1943
T. gerstaeckeri	Texas	Outside and inside	Adults	Lathrop and Ominsky, 1965; Packchanian, 1939; Wood, 1941b, 1941d
	New Mexico	Inside	Adults	Wood and Wood, 1961
	Texas	Outside	Nymphs and adults	Beard et al., 2003
T. leticularia	Texas	Inside	Nymphs and adults	Packchanian, 1940a
	South Carolina	Inside	Adults	Yabsley and Noblet, 2002a
T. protracta	Arizona	Inside	Adults	Kofoid and Whitaker, 1936; Reisenman et al., 2010; Wehrle, 1939; Wood, 1957
	Texas	Inside	Adults	Wood, 1941b
	New Mexico	Inside	Adults	Wood, 1941b
	California	Inside	Nymphs and adults	Wood, 1942a, 1950a, 1951a; Wood and Wood, 1964a
	New Mexico	Inside	Adults	Wood and Wood, 1961
	California	Inside	Nymphs and adults	Mehringer et al., 1961
	California	Inside	Adults	Sjögren and Ryckman, 1966
T. recurva	Arizona	Outside and inside	Nymphs and adults	Reisenman et al., 2010; Schuck, 1945; Wehrle, 1939; Wood, 1941a, 1941b, 1957
	California	Inside	Adults	Wood, 1955
	Texas	Outside and inside	Adults	Ikenga and Richerson, 1984
T. rubida	Arizona	Outside and inside	Nymphs and adults	Bice, 1966; Reisenman et al., 2010; Wehrle, 1939; Wood, 1941b, 1957
	Texas	Inside	Adults	Wood, 1941d
	California	Inside	Adults	Wood, 1955
T. sanguisuga	Texas	Outside and inside	Adults	Davis et al., 1943; Lathrop and Ominsky, 1965
	Kansas	Inside	Adults	Grundemann, 1947
	Texas	Inside	Adults	Elkins, 1951a; Shields and Walsh, 1956
	New Mexico	Outside and inside	Adults	Wood, 1958
	Alabama	Outside and inside	Adults	Olsen et al., 1964
		Outside and inside	Nymphs and adults	Hays, 1966
	Georgia	Outside and inside	Adults	Olsen et al., 1964
	Illinois	Inside	Nymphs and adults	Porter, 1965
	Florida	Outside and inside	Adults	Beard et al., 1988
	Louisiana	Inside	Adults	Dorn et al., 2007; Snider et al., 1980; Yaeger, 1988
	Georgia	Outside and inside	Adults	Pung et al., 1995
	Tennessee	Outside and inside	Adults*	Herwaldt et al., 2000
	South Carolina	Inside	Adults	Yabsley and Noblet, 2002

*A nymph was found in a wood pile.

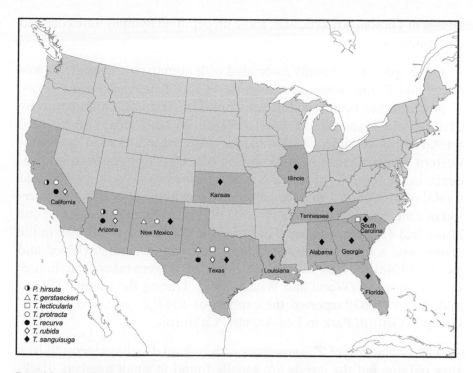

Figure 2.2. Geographic distribution of species visiting households. (See Plate 2).

We will mention a few examples of triatomines found in or around houses. Kofoid and Whitaker (1936) were the first to report the finding of *T. rubida*: 35 adult specimens in one house on two occasions, in the vicinity of Tucson, Arizona. Wehrle (1939) mentions the same species, also in Arizona, in piles of wood under homes or adjacent to chicken coops and that both nymphs and adults can be found in human dwellings. In another report, of 204 *T. rubida* captured, 109 were from houses and as many as 16 bugs were taken from one house in one night (Wood, 1941a). From three houses in Alvarado Mine, Arizona, there were 113 *T. recurva* and 34 *T. rubida*, and a woman collected 20 insects (probably *T. rubida*) from her bed on one occasion. Furthermore, there were 485 specimens of *T. rubida* and one of *T. protracta* taken from two houses in the same locality (Wood, 1941b). Also in Alvarado Mine, *T. recurva* was found in miners' houses, and in one house four bugs were taken from a bed in one night (Wood, 1941a). On another occasion, a woman found six *T. recurva* in her bed (Wood, 1941b). *T. rubida* has also been found in houses in Texas (Wood, 1941b). Reisenman et al. (2010) found 158 *T. sanguisuga* adults, five *T. recurva*, and one *T. protracta* in or around houses in Tucson, Arizona; also, some unidentified nymphs were collected inside houses.

Other species commonly associated with human dwellings are *T. protracta* and *T. sanguisuga* in several states and *T. gerstaeckeri* in Texas. *T. protracta* has been found in households in Arizona, California, New Mexico, and Texas (Wood, 1941b, 1941c). Wood (1950a) also reported a total of 144 specimens of this species collected in houses in the southwestern United States. A single person collected 15 bugs from his residence in the foothills of Sierra Nevada, California (Wood, 1950b), and a total of 44 *T. protracta* were collected in one house over a 2-month period of time, also in California (Wood, 1951a). In San Diego county, one house had 42 specimens, another house had 24 insects distributed in the rooms, and a third had 50 bugs during spring and summer (Wood and Wood, 1964a). In New Mexico, 32 *T. protracta* were taken from houses on one occasion (Wood and Wood, 1961). During the summer, Wood and Wood (1967) reported the capture of 1044 *T. protracta* at Boys' Camp in Griffith Park in Los Angeles, California.

The association of *T. sanguisuga* with human dwellings seems to be a very old one but the insects are usually found in small numbers. Packchanian (1940b) reports the finding of 50 people bitten by this insect in Sarasota, Florida, in the Civilian Conservation Corp Camps, and Porter (1965) mentions the finding of 24 adults and two nymphs inside houses in an area of Illinois. Olsen et al. (1964) mentions the collection of this species from human habitations in small towns of Alabama and Georgia. On one occasion, eight insects were found in an elderly woman's bed and a few more in the quarters of domestic animals. Hays (1966), also in Alabama, collected this species from inside seven houses; in two of them nymphs were present, and in one case nine nymphs were removed from a bed. Adults were also found in an outhouse and a doghouse, and one adult and two nymphs were found in a corn crib. Beard et al. (1988) reported a single *T. cruzi*-infected adult on the screen door of a home in Gainesville, Florida, and multiple bugs were collected inside homes in this region, where the inhabitants complained of allergic responses associated with bites. Pung et al. (1995) reported the finding of specimens of this species inside homes in Bulloch County, Georgia, and that eight bugs were collected on the wall of a storage building in the southeast of the same state. Dorn et al. (2007) collected 20 *T. sanguisuga* inside the home of an index case and in an adjacent building, and 298 additional adult insects (60.4% infected with *T. cruzi* by polymerase chain reaction demonstration) were collected over one summer inside and immediately outside the same house (Cesa et al., 2011).

As already mentioned, *T. gerstaeckeri* is another species that has been found in houses in areas of Texas. A housewife killed more than 300 specimens in 6 weeks during one summer, and more than 100 were collected on a farm; also, chickens, cows, and hogs were all reported to have been bitten by this bug (Packchanian, 1939). Beard et al. (2003) collected 31 specimens, including adults and nymphs, under cement slabs of a back porch and from a garage around a house in the community of San Benito, Texas. Packchanian (1940a) also reported the finding of more than 150 specimens of *T. lecticularia* in homes in Temple, Texas, in different areas of the city, including some nymphs that were located in beds and other parts of the houses.

2.3 INFECTION RATES OF *T. CRUZI*

Several studies have addressed the infection indices of the U.S. triatomines with *T. cruzi*, the causative agent of Chagas disease.

As previously mentioned, Kofoid and McCulloch observed the parasite for the first time in *T. protracta* in 1916 in California. In Table 2.3, we present a chronology of the records of infections by *T. cruzi* in eight species of triatomines, from 10 states, from 1916 to 2010. The distribution of the infected bugs by states is presented in Figure 2.3 (see Plate 4). The reported rates of infection, available from the literature, are shown in Table 2.4, also by species and by state. *P. hirsuta* has not been found naturally infected, but it can be infected experimentally (Wood, 1941d).

In Table 2.5, we summarize the accumulated prevalence rates, presented in Table 2.4, for the six most common species (48 specimens of *T. neotomae* are included from two reports). The table shows a total mean rate of 25.6%, which is not different from what has been reported in the most common vector species in Central and South America. Nevertheless, among the U.S. species, there are some differences, such as the observation that *T. rubida* and *T. sanguisuga* rates tend to be low, whereas the rates for *T. gerstaeckeri*, *T. lecticularia*, and *T. neotomae* (the first two species are very common in Texas) are significantly above the mean. In the case of *T. sanguisuga*, the rates vary by geography, with higher infection rates seen in Texas and Louisiana (Table 2.4).

Table 2.3. Chronological and Geographical Records of *T. cruzi* Infection in U.S. Triatomines

Species	Locality	State	References
T. protracta	San Diego	California	Kofoid and McCulloch, 1916
	Quemado Valley	Texas	De Shazo, 1943; Wood, 1941b
	Maverick Co		
	Grant	New Mexico	Wood, 1941b
	Pinal and Pima counties	Arizona	Wood, 1949
	Valverde and Uvalde	Texas	Sullivan et al., 1949
	Counties		
	Kane County	Utah	Wood, 1956
	Montezuma Castle	Arizona	Wood, 1957, 1958
	Chaco Canyon and Tyrone	New Mexico	Wood and Wood, 1961
	Counties		
	Riverside County	California	Ryckman et al., 1965
	Escondido	California	Klotz et al., 2009
	Tucson	Arizona	Klotz et al., 2009
	Several counties	Texas	Kjos et al., 2009
T. rubida	Tucson	Arizona	Kofoid and Whitaker, 1936
	Alvarado Mine and Yavapai	Arizona	Wood, 1941a; 1941b
	Counties		
	Nogales	Arizona	Schuck, 1945
	Sanderson, Terrell Co	Texas	Wood, 1941c; 1942
	Tuzigoot	Arizona	Wood, 1957, 1958
	Tucson	Arizona	Bice, 1966; Reisenman et al., 2010
T. sanguisuga	Unknown	Texas	Anonymous, 1938; Kjos et al., 2009
	Matagorda and Dimmit	Texas	Davis et al., 1943; De Shazo, 1943
	Counties		
	Several counties	Texas	Elkins, 1951a; Sullivan et al., 1949
	Lafitte-Paradis and Orleans	Louisiana	Dorn et al., 2007; Yaeger, 1961
	Several counties	Alabama	Hays et al., 1961; Olsen et al., 1964
	Cameron County	Texas	Eads et al., 1963
	Bexar County	Texas	Pippin et al., 1968
	Gainesville	Florida	Beard et al., 1988
	New Orleans	Louisiana	Dorn et al., 2007; Yaeger, 1988
	Southeast	Georgia	Pung et al., 1995
	Rutherford County	Tennessee	Herwaldt et al., 2000
T. gerstaeckeri	Three Rivers	Texas	Packchanian, 1939; Wood, 1941b; De Shazo, 1943
	Quemado Valley	Texas	Wood, 1941b
	Maverick Co		
	Sanderson	Texas	Wood, 1942a
	Several counties	Texas	Kjos et al., 2009; Sullivan et al., 1949
	Carlsbad	New Mexico	Wood and Wood, 1961
	Cameron County	Texas	Eads et al., 1963
T. lecticularia	Temple	Texas	De Shazo, 1943; Packchanian, 1940a
	Several counties	Texas	Sullivan et al., 1949; Yaeger, 1959; Kjos et al., 2009
T. recurva	Alvarado Mine	Arizona	Wood, 1941a, 1941b
	Rimrock	Arizona	Wood, 1958
	Brewster Co	*Texas*	Ikenga and Richerson, 1984
	Tucson	Arizona	Reisenman et al., 2010

Table 2.3 Chronological and Geographical Records of *T. cruzi* Infection in U.S. Triatomines—*cont'd*

Species	Locality	State	References
T. neotomae	Several counties Bandera and Cameron County	Texas Texas	De Shazo, 1943; Kjos et al., 2009 Eads et al., 1963; Sullivan et al., 1949
T. indictiva (aka *T. sanguisuga indictiva*)	Carlsbad Caverns	New Mexico	Wood, 1958

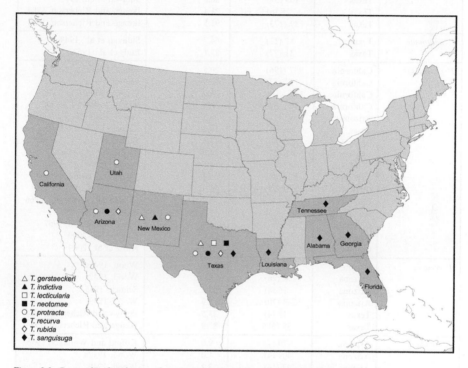

Figure 2.3. Geographic distribution of species infected with T. cruzi. (See Plate 4).

Table 2.4. *T. cruzi* Prevalence Rates in U.S. T. and Their Distribution by State

Species	State	Number Examined (Number Positive)	Infection Prevalence (%)	References
T. gerstaeckeri	Texas	100 (92)	92.0	Packchanian, 1939
	Texas	54 (3)	5.6	Wood, 1942b
	Texas	450 (135)	29.9	Sullivan et al., 1949
	N. Mexico	17 (5)	29.4	Wood and Wood, 1961
	Texas	133 (84)	63.2	Eads et al., 1963

Continued...

Table 2.4 *T. cruzi* Prevalence Rates in U.S. T. and Their Distribution by State—*cont'd*

Species	State	Number Examined (Number Positive)	Infection Prevalence (%)	References
	Texas	49 (12)	24.5	Burkholder et al., 1980
	Texas	31 (8)	25.8	Ikenga and Richerson, 1984
	Texas	31 (29)	93.7	Ikenga and Richerson, 1984
	Texas	31 (24)	77.4	Beard et al., 2003
	Texas	156 (86)	55.1	Kjos et al., 2009
T. lecticularia	Texas	150 (97)	64.7	Packchanian, 1940a
	Texas	50 (50)	100.0	Packchanian, 1940a
	Texas	109 (39)	36.6	Sullivan et al., 1949
	Texas	28 (6)	21.4	Ikenga and Richerson, 1984
	Texas	189 (173)	91.5	Ikenga and Richerson, 1984
T. neotomae	Texas	17 (11)	64.7	Sullivan et al., 1949
	Texas	31 (27)	87.1	Eads et al., 1963
T. protracta	California	957 (196)	20.5	Wood, 1941c
	California	152 (57)	37.5	Wood, 1941d
	California	816 (204)	25.0	Wood, 1942a
	California	186 (57)	30.6	Wood, 1944b
	Arizona	83 (17)	20.5	Wood, 1949
	Texas	68 (11)	16.2	Sullivan et al., 1949
	California	206 (36)	17.4	Wood, 1953b
	California	383 (92)	24.0	Mehringer and Wood, 1958
	N. Mexico	442 (18)	4.1	Wood and Wood, 1961
	California	321 (70)	21.4	Wood and Wood, 1964a
	California	170 (90)	52.9	Wood and Anderson, 1965
	California	355 (54)	15.2	Sjögren and Ryckman, 1966
	Arizona	133 (26)	19.5	Bice, 1966
	California	1759 (593)	33.7	Wood and Wood, 1967
	Arizona	4 (1)	25.0	Klotz et al., 2009
	California	20 (4)	20.0	Klotz et al., 2009
T. recurva	Arizona	62 (10)	16.1	Wood, 1941a
	Arizona	230 (26)	11.3	Wood, 1942a
	Arizona	16 (8)	50.0	Schuck, 1945
	Arizona	253 (30)	11.9	Wood, 1949
	Texas	17 (4)	23.5	Ikenga and Richerson, 1984
	Texas	58 (51)	87.9	Ikenga and Richerson, 1984
T. rubida	Arizona	79 (7)	9.0	Kofoid and Whitaker, 1936
	Arizona	407 (4)	1.0	Wood, 1942a
	Arizona	492 (16)	3.2	Wood, 1949
	Arizona	524 (39)	7.5	Bice, 1966
	Arizona	14 (0)	0.0	Klotz et al., 2009
	Arizona	158 (65)	41.1	Reisenman et al., 2010
T. sanguisuga	Florida	300 (0)	0.0	Packchanian, 1940b
	Texas	90 (23)	25.5	Sullivan et al., 1949
	Texas	226 (50)	22.1	Eads et al., 1963
	Alabama	181 (11)	6.0	Olsen et al., 1964
	Texas	35 (6)	17.1	Burkholder et al., 1980
	Texas	15 (6)	40.0	Davis et al., 1943
	Louisiana	18 (10)	55.6	Dorn et al., 2007
	Texas	29 (10)	34.5	Kjos et al., 2009

Table 2.5. Accumulated Prevalence of *T. cruzi* Infection in Seven Species of Triatomines from the United States as Derived from Table 2.4

Species	Number Examined	Number Positive	%
T. gerstaeckeri	1,052	478	45.4
T. lecticularia	546	369	67.6
T. neotomae	48	38	79.2
T. protracta	6,031	1,521	25.2
T. recurva	636	129	20.3
T. rubida	1,674	131	7.8
T. sanguisuga	894	116	12.9
Total rate	10,881	2,782	25.6

2.4 ETHOLOGY AND BIONOMICS

The close relationship between the North American triatomines and wood rats of the genus *Neotoma* was emphasized early in the 20th century by Kofoid and McCulloch (1916) and by Kofoid and Donat (1933b). Ryckman (1962), in his well-known monograph of the *T. protracta* complex, affirms that *"Triatoma* are blood-sucking ectoparasites of wood rats, *Neotoma* spp.,"* and he presents a list indicating the relationships that exist between *T. protracta* and different species of *Neotoma*. Also, by putting bugs in rat nests, Ryckman (1962) showed that the number of bugs decreased with time and that "this would seem to be rather conclusive evidence that the rat is capable of suppressing the *Triatoma* population by eating bugs when the opportunity arises." In this way, the rats probably maintain equilibrium with the bug by not allowing the colonies to grow and achieve high numbers of individuals. The eating of bugs by wood rats has also been observed by Wood (1953b). Ryckman and Ryckman (1967) demonstrated that up to three species of bugs can be found sympatric in *Neotoma* nests. *T. rubida*, *T. recurva*, and *Triatoma sinaloensis* (a Mexican species) can be found coexisting in the same den. Peterson et al. (2002) used an ecological niche model that further supported the notion of vector–host co-speciation among the Protracta species complex and their *Neotoma* hosts.

Wood (1941d) reported the finding of *P. hirsuta* associated with wood rat nests in Arizona and California; the same type of association was observed for *T. gerstaeckeri* and *T. protracta* in Texas and for the latter species in New Mexico and also for *T. rubida* in Arizona. Elkins (1951a) found numerous specimens of bugs of three species (*T. gerstaeckeri*, *T. lecticularia*, and *T. sanguisuga*) living in wood rat dens in Dallas, Denton, and Ellis counties in Texas.

Wood (1941a) points out that, from 451 wood rat nests examined, 1,303 bugs were collected, yielding an average of 2.88 bugs per nest. In another study, Wood (1944b) makes reference to 188 specimens of *T. protracta* found in 61 nests; i.e., 3.1 bugs per rat nest. Wood and Wood (1941) examined 135 wood rat nests in Arizona, New Mexico, Texas, and Utah and found 355 bugs; i.e., 2.6 bugs per nest. The largest number of bugs (*T. protracta*) found in a single nest was 85 (Wood, 1941c). Eads et al. (1963) examined 80 wood rat dens in Cameron County, Texas, and found 58 infested (72.5%) by a total of 390 bugs (6.7 bugs per nest) of three species: 226 *T. sanguisuga*, 133 *T. gerstaeckeri*, and 31 *T. neotomae*. Bice (1966) examined 153 rat dens near Tucson, Arizona, and found 657 bugs (524 *T. rubida* and 133 *T. protracta*), for an average of 4.3 bugs per den.

Even though the natural host of *T. sanguisuga* in Manhattan, Kansas, is *Neotoma floridana baileyi*, Grundemann (1947) also found that species in nests of the cotton rat *Sigmodon hispidus texanus*. Hays (1966) found an average of 4.9 bugs of this species in wood rat nests (species not mentioned) in Alabama.

In Table 2.6, we summarize the literature in relation to this association of species or subspecies of wood rats with eight species of triatomines in different U.S. states. We did not find references for *T. incrassata* and *T. recurva* in this regard, but the phenomenon probably occurs.

The natural association of wood rats with several species of triatomines has an epidemiological significance particularly in those cases where the *Neotoma* rats build their nests in attics and walls, under houses, and in close domestic proximity (Ryckman, 1981).

Another important aspect of the behavior of these bugs is that a dispersal flight of the adult insects living in *Neotoma* dens takes place during the summer, starting in May and June. During these periods, the insects have been known to invade houses in the vicinity of the dens, being attracted to lights (Wehrle, 1939; Wood, 1941c; Wood and Wood, 1964b). Apparently these insects overwinter in *Neotoma* dens as nymphs and molt to adults from May to August (Kitselman and Grundmann, 1940).

Table 2.6. Triatomines Collected in Wood Rat Nests (*Neotoma* spp.)

Species	Host	Place	References
P. hirsuta	*Neotoma lepida* *Neotoma desertorum*	California, Nevada, Arizona, California	Ryckman, 1953, 1965, 1971; Usinger, 1944; Wood, 1941d
T. gerstaeckeri	*Neotoma micropus micropus* *Neotoma sp.* *N. micropus*	Texas Texas Texas	Packchanian, 1939 Elkins, 1951b Burkholder et al., 1980; Eads et al., 1963
T. indictiva	*Neotoma sp.* *Neotoma sp.*	N. Mexico Texas	Wood, 1941c Elkins, 1951b
T. lecticularia	*Neotoma sp.* *N. micropus*	Texas Texas	Wood, 1941c Elkins, 1951b
T. neotomae	*N. micropus*	Texas	Eads et al., 1963; Elkins, 1951b
T. protracta	*N. f. macrotis* *Neotoma albigula albigula* *N. a. albigula* *N. albigula* *N. a. albigula* *Neotoma lepida lepida* *Neotoma fuscipes simplex* *N. f. annectans* *Neotoma fuscipes martirensis* *Neotoma fuscipes mohavensis* *N. l. lepida* *Neotoma lepida egressa* *Neotoma lepida grinnelli* *N. m. micropus* *Neotoma micropus canescens* *N. a. leucodon*	California California N. Mexico Texas Utah Utah California California California California California California California California California California	Kofoid and McCulloch, 1916; Ryckman et al., 1965; Wood, 1944b Wehrle, 1939 Wood, 1941c Elkins, 1951b Wood, 1941c Wood, 1941c Ryckman, 1962 Ryckman, 1962; Wood, 1941c Ryckman, 1962 Ryckman, 1962 Ryckman, 1962 Ryckman, 1962 Ryckman, 1962 Ryckman, 1962 Ryckman, 1962 Ryckman, 1962
T. rubida	*N. a. albigula* *N. albigula*	Arizona Texas	Bice, 1966; Wehrle, 1939; Wood, 1941d Elkins, 1951b
T. sanguisuga	*N. floridana baileyi* *N. floridana* *N. micropus* *Neotoma sp.* *N. micropus*	Kansas Texas Texas Alabama Texas	Grundemann, 1947 Elkins, 1951b Eads et al., 1963; Elkins, 1951b Hays et al., 1961; Hays, 1966 Burkholder et al., 1980

Wood (1941c) observed *T. rubida* and *T. recurva* in flight in Arizona, being attracted to lights, and Usinger (1944) collected the same two species in flight during the day and made reference to the collection by another person of hundreds of the insects flying to lights, also in Arizona. With a flashlight beam projected into the air at about a 45° angle, Wood (1941c) was able to spot 12 *T. rubida* and four *T. recurva* in Alvarado Mine, Arizona, as they flew across the beam. Similar behavior has been reported in southern Texas with *T. gerstaeckeri* (Beard, C.B., unpublished data) and in Louisiana with *T. sanguisuga* (Dorn, P., unpublished data).

Wood and Anderson (1965) considered that the insects have a rather short flight range with a maximum of about 1.6 km. Ryckman (1981) pointed out that some species fly on warm evenings and are attracted to lights from distances of a quarter of a mile. Sjögren and Ryckman (1966) and Ekkens (1981) stated that starvation and high temperatures are important factors in triggering the dispersal flight.

Other sylvatic habitats have also been determined for *T. sanguisuga*. Some specimens have been collected from cracks and tunnels in dead wood and inside hollow oak trees or stumps in Alabama (Olsen et al., 1964). Hays (1966) mentions finding this species commonly in Alabama in different kinds of hollow trees, with an average of 5.4 insects per infested tree. Kitselman and Grundmann (1940) found several specimens in pastures near Garrison, Kansas, where the insects were feeding upon horses. The authors reported isolating western equine encephalitis (WEE) virus from these bugs and suggested that they could be good vectors of this disease among horses, under certain circumstances. Although it is an interesting suggestion, a role for triatomines as vectors of WEE virus has never been substantiated, and the reported virus isolation was most likely an interesting phenomenon of no significance to animal or human health.

Packchanian (1940b) found that *T. sanguisuga* colonized palmetto trees (*Sabal palmetto*) in Sarasota, Florida, where they fed on tree frogs (*Hyla* sp.). Under experimental conditions, this species has been reported to accept blood from mice, rats, guinea pigs, rabbits, English sparrows, and frogs. The latter fact was confirmed by Hays (1966), who was able to feed *T. sanguisuga* on frogs and lizards in the laboratory. Wood (1944a) was also able to feed *T. recurva*, *T. rubida*, and *T. protracta* on lizards and snakes. Additionally, Porter (1965) reported two nymphs and one adult *T. sanguisuga* in the bark of a tree and a nymph in the nest of a mouse (*Peromyscus* sp.) in Illinois.

Yaeger (1961) reported finding *T. sanguisuga* in rotted, hollow trees in areas of Louisiana. Ryckman (1984) is of the opinion that, in the forested eastern areas, this species inhabits large hollow trees frequented by different mammals, independent of the *Neotoma* rats as a source of blood and habitat. Furthermore, he believes that *T. sanguisuga* exhibits considerable adaptability to different ecological niches over a distance of 2,500 km, from southwestern Texas to south central Florida (Ryckman, 1986).

Packchanian (1949) reported an association of *T. lecticularia* with armadillo and opossum nests. Elkins (1951a) makes reference to observations of *T. gerstaeckeri* and *T. sanguisuga* on the ground in sparsely wooded areas and the latter species also in sweepings of tree foliage. Elkins (1951b) adds dog kennels, chicken houses, and stalls of horses and cattle as places where *T. sanguisuga* can be found, the dog kennel being confirmed by Nieto et al. (2009).

Due to their habit of visiting households, some species can be found commonly in peridomiciliary habitats. Wehrle (1939) reported finding *T. rubida* in piles of wood under houses and in adjacent poultry houses, and Wood (1950a) observed *T. protracta* in lumber piles near homes. *T. protracta* and *T. gerstaeckeri* have been found in cobwebs and chicken houses (Wood, 1941b). *T. gerstaeckeri* has also been seen in barns and *T. lecticularia* in chicken huts (Packchanian, 1939).

In relation to the life cycle of the North American species of triatomines, some, such as *P. hirsuta* and *T. recurva*, require two full years to complete the life cycle from egg to adult, while other species, such as *T. rubida*, *T. lecticularia*, *T. gerstaeckeri*, and *T. protracta*, have a 1-year life cycle (Usinger, 1944). The process, however, is dependent on temperature (Ryckman, 1962). Thurman (1944), starting with a few eggs from a single female of *T. neotomae*, observed that the incubation period was 21 days and that the first adult emerged 1 year and 27 days after the first eggs were laid. Pippin (1970) made some biological observations of two North American species, *T. sanguisuga* and *T. gerstaeckeri*, and compared them with *R. prolixus*, a very efficient vector of Chagas disease in some countries. The life cycle of *T. sanguisuga* outdoors takes 24–30 months and that of *T. gerstaeckeri* takes 9–14 months. Pippin also presented information on fecundity and number of eggs produced, longevity of adults, developmental periods of all nymphal stages, defecation and feeding times, and amount of blood ingested for the three species. A female of *T. sanguisuga* had a life span of 813 days and deposited 1,066 eggs in that period.

Hays (1965) conducted studies on fecundity, longevity, fertility, and food consumption of adults of *T. sanguisuga*. Starting with a group of nine females, obtained from field nymphs, he observed that these females laid an average of 711 eggs with a minimum of 312 and a maximum of 1,166. From a total of 5,925 eggs, the incubation period was 21–26 days at 25°C at a relative humidity of 88–93%. Hatching varied from 54 to 89% (mean: 77%), and the life span was 251–609 days (mean: 456.5 days) for females and 345–679 days (mean: 526 days) for males. The total blood consumed during adulthood varied from 2,191 to 8,349 mg for the females (mean: 5,377 mg) and from 1,880 to 4,721 mg for the males (mean: 3,488 mg). In the same species, Hays (1966) found that eggs hatched in the range of 21–33°C with an optimum hatching temperature of 26°C. Eggs did not hatch at low humidity. The optimal humidity range was 65–92%. Similarly, nymphs subjected to a relative humidity below 65% lived only up to 9 days. Eggs kept at 21°C required 39–44 days to hatch, whereas those kept at 33°C hatched in 16–18 days.

Thurman (1945a) presented similar data for *T. gerstaeckeri* and stated that females could lay a mean of 245.4 eggs per female over their entire lives with the life cycle requiring from 190 to 250 days under optimal laboratory conditions. The life span of adults ranged from 6 to 11 months. He also observed that the nymphal life span could be greatly extended as a result of adverse conditions.

Ryckman (1962) studied several reproductive parameters of *T. protracta* and its "subspecies" and of *T. rubida*. For *T. protracta*, the mean number of eggs per female was 243.2, and for *T. rubida* it was 466.5. He also studied the starvation capacity of *T. protracta* nymphs and adults, showing that they can endure fasting from 3 to 4 months as small nymphs and adults and from 7 to 10 months as larger nymphs. The life span of *T. protracta* adults can vary from a maximum of 223 days for females to 568 days for males, whereas the life spans of *T. rubida* were 276 and 204 days, respectively. Thurman (1945b) reported the amount of blood taken by each of the five nymphal instars of *T. gerstaeckeri*. Also, Wood (1959) measured the amount of blood ingested by the different nymphal instars and by the adults of *T. protracta*, *T. rubida*, *T. recurva*, and *P. hirsuta*. In another paper, Wood (1942a) reported the engorgement time of adults of five species of triatomines and found that the smallest species, *P. hirsuta*, takes 6.3–11.5 minutes for repletion; the three medium-sized species, *T. rubida*, *T. protracta*, and *T. sanguisuga*, take 8–11.5, 11.5–12.5, and 24–30 minutes, respectively; and the largest species of this group, *T. gerstaeckeri*, takes approximately 15.5 minutes.

The amount of blood ingested by nymphs and adults and the resistance to fasting were studied by Jurberg and Costa (1989) for *T. lecticularia*. Fifth-instar nymphs resisted periods of starvation for longer, with the time ranging from 48 to 238 days (average: 162.3 days).

The male genital structures of *T. rubida*, *T. gerstaeckeri*, *T. lecticularia*, *T. protracta*, *T. recurva*, *T. rubida*, and *T. sanguisuga* were described in detail by Lent and Jurberg (1987). Also, Rocha et al. (1996) did morphological and morphometric studies of eggs and nymphs of *T. lecticularia*.

In Table 2.7, we present data on the life cycles of some North American species according to the literature. When compared with *R. prolixus*, Pipping (1970) came to the conclusion that *T. sanguisuga* and *T. gerstaeckeri* are more timid in attacking the victim and that the percentage of defecation is much higher for *R. prolixus*. Nevertheless, around one-fourth of the fourth and fifth nymph instars and adult females of *T. sanguisuga* and *T. gerstaeckeri* were able to defecate within 2 minutes of feeding, making them better fecal contaminants than the other stages and consequently good potential vectors.

Wood (1943) found that *T. recurva* is much slower in its feeding and moving reactions than *T. rubida*. He also pointed out that *T. protracta*, *T. recurva*, and *P. hirsuta* are slow defecators and that *T. rubida* is faster. For *T. protracta*, the time of defecation was 0.1–133 minutes, and four specimens did not defecate between 89 and 223 minutes of a blood meal, whereas *T. rubida* was more efficient, with a defecation time ranging between 0.1 and 6 minutes (Wood, 1951b). Wood (1960), in a more detailed report, presented the mean time for the first defecation for each of the nymphal stages and for the adults of *T. protracta*, indicating a range from 22.2 to 59.5 minutes, with some nymphs defecating more than the adults, but still making this species a very slow defecator and potentially a poor vector of Chagas disease.

Nogueda-Torres et al. (2000) have described the defecation patterns of seven species of triatomines from Mexico, including *T. lecticularia*, concluding that this species "may be considered as highly efficient vectors of *T. cruzi*," close to *R. prolixus* and *T. infestans*. A similar conclusion was drawn by Martínez-Ibarra et al. (2005) in relation to the Mexican *T. rubida* (*T. rubida sonoriana*). By observing the defecation times of the different nymphal instars and adult stages, they concluded that all, except the males, acted as efficient defecators.

Table 2.7. Life Cycle of Some North American Species of Triatomines as Presented by Some Authors

Species	Mean of Days in Each Instar						Mean Life Span		Total (from egg to adult)	T/RH	References
	Egg	I	II	III	IV	V	Male	Female			
T. gerstaeckeri	16	20	25	42	48	90	-	-	241	RT	Thurman, 1945a
T. gerstaeckeri	26.4	53.2	27.4	68.2	107.1	79.6	285.4	285.0	361.9	18-30/20-65	Pippin, 1970
T. gerstaeckeri	17.1	14.8	15.7	17.3	71.3	77.7	317.4	312.6	213.9	27/65	Pippin, 1970
T. gerstaeckeri	22.7	22.6	21.8	41.8	59.3	97.9	-	-	278.6	27/30	Martinez-Ibarra et al., 2007
T. protracta	20.8	16.0	18.2	22.1	24.5	31.6	136.8	129.1	133.2	29/50	Ryckman, 1962
T. protracta	19.2	34.6	49.6	54.0	64.6	70.5	-	-	269.6	27/30	Martinez-Ibarra et al., 2007
T. sanguisuga	23.6	53.4	46.1	72.8	126.6	65.3	527.4	589.2	387.8	18-30/20-65	Pippin, 1970
T. sanguisuga	22.8	28.6	37.8	61.8	84.8	85.3	625.6	516.4	322.1	27/65	Pippin, 1970
T. rubida (T. r. sonoriana)	16.3	12.8	14.1	17.8	23.3	33.3	-	-	119.7	27/70	Martinez-Ibarra et al., 2005
T. lecticularia	18.9	29.2	54.1	58.6	44.2	67.8	-	-	234.9	27/30	Martinez-Ibarra et al., 2007

Note: T, temperature (°C); RH, relative humidity (%); RT, room temperature.

In the study by Martínez-Ibarra et al. (2007), using specimens of *T. gerstaeckeri, T. lecticularia,* and *T. protracta* from Mexico, different biological parameters were measured for the three species. Eclosion rates and incubation periods of the eggs, the entire life cycle, mortality rates, mean number of blood meals between instars and feeding, and defecation times were compared. The developmental time from egg to adult was shorter for *T. lecticularia,* and it took from about 8 to 9 months in all species. Postfeeding defecation times were less than 10 minutes for younger nymphs of *T. gerstaeckeri* and for all instars of *T. lecticularia* and *T. protracta,* making them potentially effective vectors.

Klotz et al. (2009) also studied the feeding and defecation patterns of adult *T. protracta* and *T. rubida* from the southwestern United States. They reported that *T. rubida* initiated feeding slightly faster than *T. protracta* (within 2.3 vs. 4 minutes) and that *T. rubida* fed longer than *T. protracta* (27.9 vs. 22.8 minutes), and that the amount of blood ingested per meal was greatest for *T. rubida* females, followed by *T. protracta* females, *T. rubida* males, and then *T. protracta* males. On the basis of the defecation patterns, they concluded that the two species would be poor vectors of Chagas disease in that region. This suggests, in the case of *T. rubida,* some differences in defecation times between insects from different geographical regions. This variation in behavior might be explained by phylogenetic differences among populations of the so-called rubida complex, which, according to certain authors, involves more than one species and several subspecies (Adams and Ryckman, 1969; Ibarra-Cerdeña et al., 2009; Pfeiler et al., 2006).

A phenomenon common in triatomine bugs, observed for the first time by Brumpt (1914) and called cannibalism, was noticed by Ryckman (1951) in *T. recurva* nymphs. By this mechanism, a younger nymph can suck blood or hemolymph from a larger companion, and this prompted Ryckman to propose the term "cleptohemodeipnonism" (stolen blood) for the phenomenon. Hays (1965) points out that, through cannibalism, one first instar nymph of *T. sanguisuga* reached the fourth nymphal stage and that the process is used as a mechanism of survival by the early-stage nymphs. Hays (1966) also made reference to this phenomenon as the ability of *T. sanguisuga* nymphs to feed on hemolymph of other insects and reported that one insect was maintained in the laboratory for 556 days solely on hemolymph.

2.5 ALLERGIC REACTIONS TO KISSING BUG BITES

The first records of discomfort and allergic reactions caused by triatomine bites in people were reported in the 19th century. Le Conte (1855) made reference to *T. sanguisuga* bites in Georgia that were followed by "very serious consequences." Similar observations were made in Kansas by Kimball (1894), who described severe local reactions at the site of the bite extending to other parts of the body and systemic reactions such as severe headache and nausea followed by depression. Howard (1899), referring to the same species in Missouri, claimed that its bite produced intense itching and swelling lasting 3–4 days. Both Le Conte (1855) and Howard (1899) affirmed that the reactions produced by the kissing bugs were commonly and unjustly attributed by people to spider bites.

Ryley and Howard (1894) made reference to the case of a woman from Arizona with systemic reactions following the bite of an unidentified *Triatoma* (*T. protracta*?). Morrill (1914) stated that in southwest Arizona there was "a blood-sucking cone-nosed bug belonging to the genus *Conorhinus*, which is quite troublesome as a home hold pest" and capable of producing "red blotches and welts all over the body and limbs." This blood sucker of Arizona was referred to as *C. sanguisugus* (*T. sanguisuga*) by Morrill but may have been a different species (Ryckman, 1984).

Kofoid and Whitaker (1936) mentioned a person in Tucson, Arizona, who became sensitized following several *T. rubida* bites and displayed both local and systemic reactions; they pointed out that subsequent bites "result[ed] in desensitization, the reaction becoming less and less severe." Wehrle (1939) also made reference to "severe reactions" resulting from the bites of *T. rubida* in Arizona.

Africa (1934) reported the first three adult cases of allergic and anaphylactic reactions to the bites of the cosmopolitan species *T. rubrofasciata* in the Philippine Islands, with general symptoms and local manifestations. Similarly, Arnold and Bell (1944) found two cases of local reactions in Hawaii, where this species has resided since its purported introduction near the beginning of the 20th century. *T. rubrofasciata* seems to be common in certain areas close to Honolulu. Teo and Cheah (1973) described a severe anaphylactic reaction in a 19-year-old man caused by the bite of *T. rubrofasciata* in Singapore.

Wood (1941b) contributed to the knowledge of the signs and symptoms of the allergic and anaphylactic reactions of individuals to triatomine bites after becoming acquainted with this phenomenon in Arizona. He studied his own reaction to bites he sustained under progressive experimental conditions. He felt no physical discomfort and experienced a local irritation only with a single species, *P. hirsuta* (Wood, 1942a). In an area of Sierra Nevada, California, where *T. protracta* is a common visitor, he observed reactions to the bites in several people including severe itching over the body, edema, nausea, diarrhea, and dizziness; one person also became unconsciousness for a few hours (Wood, 1950b). A similar picture was also observed at Griffith Park, Los Angeles, California, produced by the same species, and in Arizona and New Mexico, produced by *T. protracta* and *T. rubida* bites (Wood, 1953a, 1953b).

Shields and Walsh (1956) characterized the local reactions to triatomine bites in a group of 45 patients who sought medical care over a 2-year period in Forth Worth, Texas, because of dermatologic lesions produced by the bite of *T. sanguisuga*. Patients came from all types of dwellings and all economic levels and all were able to find the insect in or around their beds. The bites were more frequent from April to November. They were painless, and the severity of the reactions depended on sensitization from previous bites. The authors divided the types of reactions into four main groups, primarily to familiarize dermatologists with the clinical picture that may result from the bite of these insects. The first group included papular lesions with a central punctum, sometimes resembling an atypical herpes zoster. The second group presented with small vesicles, moderate swelling, and little redness, similar to contact dermatitis. The third group displayed giant urticarial-type lesions, with firm wheals, generally erythematous, with brawny edema. The fourth and final group presented with hemorrhagic nodular-to-bullows lesions on the hands or feet similar to unilateral erythema multiforme. Lymphangytis and lymphadenitis were occasionally present in the last two groups. Those who had previous bites had more severe reactions.

Walsh and Jones (1962) stated that "the medical and social importance of reactions to the bites is becoming generally recognized and is probably greater than is presently assumed." They conducted an epidemiologic survey in the Sierra Nevada foothills, California, in 110 people with a history of being bitten by *T. protracta*. Some had local cutaneous reactions, and 84% had some type of systemic reaction, with 29%

requiring hospitalization. The signs and symptoms, in order of descending frequency, were pruritus (86%), edema mainly around the eyes, tongue, larynx, and trachea (72%), difficulty in speaking, breathing, and swallowing (51%), welts and rashes (50%), nausea (42%), fainting (32%), pain (29%), vomiting (25%), fever (24%), cramps (20%), and diarrhea (17%). Some of the symptoms seen less frequently include dizziness, palpitation, memory loss, malaise, body aches, and weakness. These authors claim that most people do not react to the bites, and there is evidence to suggest that the reactions initially are mild and later on become more severe and systemic.

Swezey (1963) reported a case of systemic reaction to the bite of *T. protracta* in a 35-year-old woman from Benedict Canyon, a region of Beverly Hills, California. Nichols and Green (1963) also carried out studies in the Sierra Nevada area and observed that 12 patients presented with an immediate positive skin test reaction to an antigen made of an extract of *T. protracta*. Wolf (1969) related that there were "numerous patients" sensitive to *Triatoma* bites seen in Temple, Texas. Four of those with severe reactions were desensitized with an extract made from the bodies of the insects but refused test bites to prove it. Lynch and Pinnas (1978), while describing some allergic cases from near Tucson, Arizona, made reference to vaginal bleeding, among other manifestations of the systemic reaction, in several patients. Topical steroids are recommended for local reactions, and for anaphylactic accidents immediate therapy with epinephrine and antihistamines is required (Lynch and Pinnas, 1978). Pinnas et al. (1978) prepared body extracts from insects, which were assayed for enzyme activity, histamine release, and production of specific IgE antibodies. The saliva was reported to contain hyaluronidase and other proteins for which specific reactions could be identified in patients receiving skin tests.

Ryckman (1981) claimed that 5–15% of people who are bitten develop some degree of hypersensitivity and that the reactions are produced by the bites of *T. protracta*, *T. recurva*, *T. rubida*, and *P. hirsuta* in California, Nevada, Arizona, Colorado, and New Mexico. He exposed 495 young adults to the bite of a single specimen of four species of triatomines and observed moderate skin reactions in only 2.5% of this group, who could have been previously sensitized, even though the subjects had no history of prior exposure to triatomine bites (Ryckman, 1985). Ryckman (1979) and Ryckman and Bentley (1979) have published, in two parts, a literature review and annotated bibliography on "host reactions to bug bites." In the first paper, Ryckman (1979) makes reference to an autopsy (an unpublished report) of a person who died with acute laryngeal edema and severe pulmonary congestion and edema, caused by hypersensitivity to the bite of *T. protracta.*

Marshall and Street (1982) noted that an increasing number of cases of allergic reaction to triatomine bites are being recognized and that they can represent a seasonal annoyance or a real threat, depending on the degree of sensitization of the individuals. One factor these authors considered to be of epidemiologic importance, leading to an increase in *Triatoma*–human contact, is the development of rural areas and the spread of suburbs into previously undisturbed areas where the bugs have been living over previous decades. They described a case with a severe reaction who successfully received immunotherapy with a *T. protracta* salivary gland extract. The allergy was shown to be an IgE-mediated hypersensitivity, and, after the progressive subcutaneous injection of the antigen, the IgE levels decreased, and the patient tolerated well a *Triatoma* bite challenge on day 362 of the immunotherapy.

Rohr et al. (1984) developed a more systematic and successful immunotherapy program for *T. protracta*-induced anaphylaxis. They selected patients with histories of life-threatening allergic reactions and elevated pretreatment IgE anti-*Triatoma* antibody levels. All patients responded satisfactorily to the immunotherapy regimen they developed, and after several weeks none of the patients developed systemic reactions to a bite challenge by the insect.

Marshall et al. (1986) performed an epidemiologic survey on the prevalence of IgE antibodies to *T. protracta* salivary antigens, in a representative population at risk in Santa Barbara County, California. They found that 6.7% of the 170 people tested had elevated levels of IgE-specific antibodies. On the basis of the data obtained, they estimated that there were 30,000 people at potential risk of serious reactions, with significant elevated IgE levels to *T. protracta* antigens, in California alone. The authors also showed that there is no cross-reactivity between *T. protracta* and other triatomine antigens. Similarly, Pinnas et al. (1986) measured specific IgE in sensitized patients, by using a radioactive test (RAST), in the presence of gland extracts from *T. protracta* and *T. rubida*, showing that sensitization is species specific.

Chapman et al. (1986) isolated two protein fractions of 18,000–20,000 daltons from the salivary glands of *T. protracta* that contained most of the allergenic activity of this species. Paddock et al. (2001) have reported the purification and cloning of procalin, a lipocalin family protein considered to be the major allergenic protein of the salivary glands of *T. protracta*. Lipocalin-based proteins with antihemostatic properties have been isolated from the salivary glands of *Triatoma pallidipennis* and *R. prolixus* and are major allergens of other insects and animals. These authors suggest that procalin be used in serological testing to identify people at risk for which desensitization may be useful to reduce the risk of severe allergic reactions to the bite of *T. protracta*.

Moffitt et al. (2003) reviewed some aspects of the problems associated in the United States with allergic reactions to the bites of these insects and summarized some of the technical knowledge in relation to the geographical distribution of the five species commonly involved, the types of reactions and *Triatoma* allergens, the management of the clinical picture, and the immunological profiles of the patients. Another review by Goddard (2003) presents a more general picture of the problem, focusing mainly on the public health aspect.

More recently, Klotz et al. (2010) made reference to the different types of reactions produced after triatomine bites in the United States. They presented four cases of allergic reactions: one in a 46-year-old woman from San Diego, California, with a diagnosis of anaphylaxis, produced from the bite of a *T. protracta*; and two in women aged 57 and 37 years, from Louisiana and Arizona, respectively, with "false Romaña's signs," after being bitten on their faces by *T. sanguisuga* in the first case and by *T. rubida* in the second case. The other patient, a 63-year-old woman from Arizona, showed a localized swelling, and she was able to find specimens of *T. rubida* and *T. recurva* where she was living.

From what is found in the literature on these allergic and anaphylactic reactions to triatomine bites, we can infer that there is a marked contrast in what is reported in the United States and what occurs in Latin America. Although in the United States the reactions have been known for more than a century and are commonly observed in certain areas, sometimes with serious consequences, and seem to be an increasing public health problem, this is not the case in Latin America, where the reports of these reactions have been infrequent and sporadic.

Medical entomology or parasitology textbooks from the United States frequently make reference to this problem, whereas Latin American books fail to mention the phenomenon as a public health concern. Occasional reports from Latin America, however, constitute evidence that this is an uncommon phenomenon among people who live in endemic areas of Chagas disease and that serious systemic reactions very rarely occur and in some areas may be completely lacking.

Balazuc (1950) reported his own experience after allowing *T. infestans* nymphs to bite him periodically and, as a consequence, becoming sensitized, leading to systemic anaphylactic reactions. The process was reversed, however, through a subsequent series of bites that resulted in desensitization and mild reactions. Zeledón (1953), while describing a local and generalized reaction in a patient submitted to xenodiagnosis with *Triatoma dimidiata* nymphs, noticed that the reaction was specific and was not produced or was less severe when other species of bugs, such as *Rhodnius pallescens* or *T. infestans*, were used. An accidental case was reported by Lapierre and Lariviere (1954) in a woman who took care of laboratory colonies of *R. prolixus* and suffered anaphylactic shock as a consequence of periodic bites.

Dias (1968) made the observation that no serious reactions were observed in humans exposed to triatomine bites in endemic regions of Brazil. Even after numerous xenodiagnoses were performed on these people, the majority had only local weak allergic reactions, and more than one-third had no reactions at all. Again, the intensity of the local reactions could be related to the species of triatomine involved. Similar observations were made by Costa et al. (1981) while using xenodiagnosis with specimens of *T. infestans* and *D. maxima* in an area of Brazil where the former species was the local domestic vector.

Maekelt (1974) reported cutaneous allergic reactions in people from Venezuela who were field tested by xenodiagnosis, with 40–80 or more specimens of *R. prolixus*. The hypersensitivity reactions were not observed when using *T. infestans*. On the other hand, Mott et al. (1980) observed the same type of allergic reactions 48–72 hours after the application of xenodiagnosis with *T. infestans*, in people from a rural area of Brazil where *P. megistus* was the only domestic vector. The authors suggest that either a reaction to the saliva of *T. infestans* without previous sensitization or a cross-reaction in persons previously sensitized to the saliva of *P. megistus* may explain this phenomenon. It has been shown that the protein composition of the saliva of these two species share four fractions, out of 24 and 19, respectively (Pereira et al., 1996). If this could explain, the cross-reactivity observed by Mott et al. (1980) would have to be demonstrated.

A study by Nascimento et al. (2001) found that humans, including patients with Chagas disease, living in endemic areas infested by the domiciliary species *T. infestans* had elevated levels of antibodies of the subclasses IgG1 and IgG4 against the proteins of the salivary glands of that species, but the levels of IgE of all groups studied were very low. They mentioned that "IgG4 serum levels might serve as an indicator of intensity of exposure to insect bites." This finding prompted Moffitt et al. (2003) to speculate that this might be the reason "why there are no frequent reports of allergic reactions from these areas."

It needs to be evaluated whether the relative absence of these systemic anaphylactic reactions in Latin America could be due to qualitative differences in allergenicity between United States and Latin American species of triatomines or due to quantitative proportions of the responsible antigens in the salivary glands. One feasible hypothesis is that the anaphylactic incidents in the United States are more frequent in people who are exposed to the bites of insects rarely, e.g., once a year, or when insects visit homes or campgrounds during the summers, leading to easier sensitization. This may not be the case in Latin America, where people are regularly exposed to the bites of insects that colonize their homes. In the latter case, the people who live in endemic areas are prone to becoming desensitized due to constant bites received throughout the year.

Nevertheless, we have to keep in mind some possible differences between the proteins and other substances in the salivary glands of these bugs. Ribeiro et al. (1998) noticed qualitative differences between species in the pattern of apyrase activation by divalent cations, and smooth muscle active compounds were also qualitatively distinct. Furthermore, *T. protracta, T. lecticularia*, and *T. picturata* have potent vasodilators both in the presence and in the absence of endothelium, whereas in *Triatoma* species from South America the vasodilators are endothelium dependent.

CHAPTER 3

Animal Reservoirs

3.1 WILD RESERVOIRS

Several wild mammals have been found to be naturally infected with *T. cruzi* in the United States (Tables 3.1 and 3.2 and Figure 3.1, see Plate 5). The first reported was a wood rat (*N. fuscipes macrotis*) from Murray Canyon, near San Diego, California (Wood, 1934). The same rat was later confirmed to be infected in California (Wood 1952a; Wood, 1975; Wood and Hughes, 1953).

In Texas, Packchanian (1942) found one of 15 armadillos (*D. novem-cinctus*) eight of eight opossums, two of two house mice, and 32 of 100 wood rats (*N. m. micropus*) examined to be infected with *T. cruzi*. Amastigotes were found in the heart of the infected wood rats. Wood (1949) added *N. a. albigula* and *Peromyscus boylii rowleyi* from Arizona to the list of animals infected, along with *Peromyscus truei gilberti* from California (Wood, 1952a). Wood (1952b) also discussed the report of *T. cruzi*-infected bats in the country, coming to the conclusion that they are parasitized by *T. vespertilionis*, a closely related species.

The first report of raccoons infected with *T. cruzi* was that of Walton et al. (1956), who found three infected animals at the Patuxent Research Refuge in Laurel, Maryland.

Brooke et al. (1957) found one skunk, one raccoon, and several opossums infected in the state of Georgia. McKeever et al. (1958) found 93 of 552 opossums (*Didelphis marsupialis*), two of 118 gray foxes (*Urocyon cinereoargenteus*), nine of 608 raccoons, and three of 306 infected striped skunks (*Mephitis mephitis*) in southwestern Georgia and northwestern Florida to be infected. McKeever et al. (1958) isolated *T. cruzi* from the urine of infected opossums and suggested that other transmission methods, including through contaminated urine, may explain the high incidence of infection in this animal. Yaeger (1971) showed in the laboratory that opossums may become infected while eating infected bugs.

An Appraisal of the Status of Chagas Disease in the United States. DOI: 10.1016/B978-0-12-397268-2.00003-1

Table 3.1. Wild Animal Reservoirs of *T. cruzi*, by Parasite Demonstration, Reported Chronologically in the United States by State

Common Name	Scientific Name	State	References
San Diego wood rat	*N. fuscipes*	California	Wood, 1934b, 1952a; Wood and Hughes, 1953
Armadillo	*Dasypus novemcinctus texanus*	Texas, Louisiana	Barr et al., 1991a; Packchanian, 1942; Yaeger, 1988
House mouse	*Mus musculus*	Texas	Packchanian, 1942
Southern plains wood rat	*N. m. micropus*	Texas	Burkholder et al., 1980; Packchanian, 1942
White-throated wood rat	*N. a. albigula*	Arizona, New Mexico	Wood, 1949; Wood and Wood, 1961
Deer mouse	*P. b. rowleyi*	Arizona	Wood, 1949
White-footed mouse	*P. t. gilberti*	California	Wood, 1952a
Striped skunk	*Mephitis mephitis*	Georgia, Florida, California	Brooke et al., 1957; McKeever et al., 1958; Ryan et al., 1985
Gray fox	*Urocyon cinereoargenteus*	Georgia, Florida	McKeever et al., 1958
Antelope squirrel	*Ammospermophilus leucurus cinnamoneus*	New Mexico	Wood and Wood, 1961
Southern plain wood rat	*N. m. canescens*	New Mexico	Wood and Wood, 1961
Western harvest mouse	*Reithrodontomys megalotis*	California	Wood, 1962
Ring-tail cat	*Bassariscus astutus*	Texas	Kagan et al., 1966; Lathrop and Ominsky, 1965
White-footed mouse	*P. truei montipinoris*	California	Wood, 1975
Pocket mouse	*Perognathus hispidus*	Texas	Burkholder et al., 1980
Grasshopper mouse	*Onychomys leucogaster*	Texas	Burkholder et al., 1980
Pocket mouse	*Liomys irroratus*	Texas	Burkholder et al., 1980
California ground squirrel	*Spermophilus beecheyi*	California	Navin et al., 1985

It is worth noting that Deane et al. (1984) have shown that *T. cruzi* can be directly transmitted by opossums (*D. marsupialis*). The insect's infectious stages (metacyclic trypanosomes) are present in the lumen of the anal glands of experimentally and naturally infected opossums (Deane et al., 1984; Fernandes et al., 1987; Steindel et al., 1987).

Habermann et al. (1958) and Walton et al. (1958) also reported infected raccoons in Maryland. Parasites were observed in fresh blood, and amastigotes were found in the cardiac muscle (Walton et al., 1958). Herman and Bruce (1962), while examining 2,005 mammals of 18 species, collected at the Patuxent Wildlife Research Center in Maryland,

Table 3.2. Raccoons and Opossums Found Naturally Infected with *T. cruzi* in the United States, Reported by State

Common Name	Scientific Name	State	References
Opossum	*D. virginiana* and/or *D. marsupialis*	Texas	Eads et al., 1963; Packchanian, 1942
		Arizona	Packchanian, 1942
		Georgia	Broke et al., 1957; McKeever et al., 1958; Olsen et al., 1964; Pung et al., 1995
		Florida	McKeever et al., 1958
		Alabama	Hays et al., 1961; Olsen et al., 1964
		Louisiana	Barr et al., 1991a
		North Carolina	Karsten et al., 1992
Raccoon	*Procyon lotor*	Maryland	Habermann et al., 1958; Herman and Bruce, 1962; Walton et al., 1956, 1958
		Georgia	Brooke et al., 1957; McKeever et al., 1958; Pietrzak and Pung, 1998; Pung et al., 1995; Schaffer et al., 1978; Yabsley et al., 2001
		Florida	McKeever et al., 1958; Schaffer et al., 1978; Telford and Forrester, 1991
		Louisiana	Yaeger and D´Alessandro-Bacigalupo, 1960
		Alabama	Olsen et al., 1964
		Texas	Schaffer et al., 1978
		Oklahoma	John and Hoppe, 1986
		North Carolina	Karsten et al., 1992
		Tennessee	Herwaldt et al., 2000

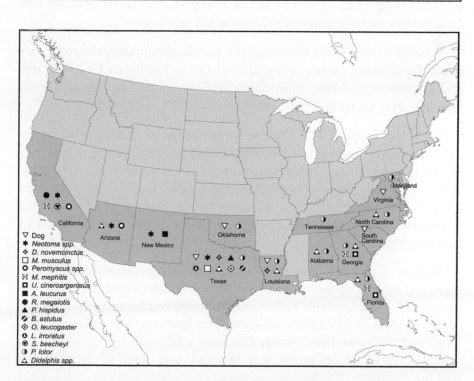

Figure 3.1. Geographic distribution of known T. cruzi animal reservoirs. (See Plate 5).

observed 10 of 472 raccoons to be infected with *T. cruzi*. Eads et al. (1963) made reference to 63 positive opossums, detected by fresh blood examination, out of 391 examined in Texas. Olsen et al. (1964) examined 181 mammals trapped in east-central Alabama, representing seven different species, and found 17 of 126 opossums and five of 35 raccoons to be infected. In one opossum the parasite was isolated from the urine, in another five opossums and in one raccoon the parasite was isolated from the peritoneal fluid, and in most cases the parasite was isolated from either the blood or the heart and kidney tissues.

Wood and Wood (1961) and Wood (1962) reported an infected squirrel (*A. l. cinnamoneus*) and an infected wood rat (*N. a. albigula*), both from New Mexico, and an infected mouse (*R. megalotis*) from California. Kagan et al. (1966) added the ring-tailed cat (*B. astutus*) to the list and another species of wood rat (*N. l. lepida*), without mentioning the places where they were found infected. The only other reference to the ring-tailed cat is that of Lathrop and Ominsky (1965) in Texas, but it is not clear if this animal was really found infected. Three new rodents were found infected by Burkholder et al. (1980) in Texas: two pocket mice (*P. hispidus* and *L. irroratus*) and one grasshopper mouse (*O. leucogaster*).

Schaffer et al. (1978) discussed the translocation and release of raccoons for hunting purposes throughout the southeastern United States and the finding of four infected individuals from Florida, five from Georgia, and six from Texas, from a total of 94 examined.

John and Hope (1986) reviewed the species of mammals naturally infected with *T. cruzi* and reported the first infected raccoons (five out of eight) from Tulsa, Oklahoma. Almost at the same time, Fox et al. (1986) detected five *T. cruzi*-infected raccoons trapped near an area where a dog had been found infected, also in Oklahoma. Telford and Forrester (1991) found two infected raccoons out of 184 examined in two counties of Florida.

Barr et al. (1991a) examined 48 opossums (16 positive by blood cultures and two more by histology) and 98 armadillos (only one positive by culture) from southern Louisiana and observed histological evidence of myocarditis in 22 of the opossums. The first report of infected opossums and raccoons from North Carolina was made by Karsten et al. (1992). One of 12 opossums was infected, and three of 20 raccoons had the parasite.

In another survey, in southeast Georgia, Pung et al. (1995) found six of 39 opossums and 12 of 54 raccoons examined to be infected with *T. cruzi*. In addition, Pietrzak and Pung (1998) reported 13 out of 30 raccoons trapped on St. Catherines Island, Georgia, to be infected, and observed amastigotes of the parasite in the heart of one animal.

By comparing IFAT and ELISA serological tests with blood cultures for the detection of raccoons infected with *T. cruzi* in southeast Georgia, Yabsley et al. (2001) found a 96% sensitivity of the two tests in detecting the 25 culture-positive samples (the serology failed only in one sample) out of 83 animals examined. The combination of both serological tests detected 42 infected animals (84%) out of 50 seropositive raccoons by either IFAT or ELISA tests. Of the 58 culture-negative animals, 19 (33%) were seropositive with both tests. In St. Catherines Island, both IFAT and ELISA detected a prevalence of 65% of the trapped raccoons infected with *T. cruzi*. Serological infections in raccoons in South Carolina have also been reported by Yabsley and Noblet (2002a). Of 181 sera samples tested by IFAT, 87 (48%) were seropositive. Similar observations have been reported from raccoons evaluated from an urban area in Fairfax County, Virginia, where 154 of 464 (32.2%) displayed anti-*T. cruzi* antibodies (Hancock et al., 2005). In Table 3.3, we have summarized some data related to the infection rates, by demonstration of the parasite, in opossums and raccoons, in different states. By using an indirect hemagglutination test, a *T. cruzi* antibody prevalence averaging 39% was found in Louisiana in 415 armadillos trapped during a 4-year study (Paige et al., 2002).

Some other wild animals have been examined by serology. Burkholder et al. (1980), using the indirect hemagglutination test (IHA), were able to demonstrate antibodies against *T. cruzi* in 20 out of 156 (12.8%) coyotes (*Canis latrans*) and in two badgers (*Taxidea taxus*) out of eight (25%) examined in the lower Rio Grande Valley of Texas. Grögl et al. (1984), also in Texas, and using the IFAT test as the serological method, found 19 coyotes out of 134 examined to be infected (14.2%).

Rosypal et al. (2007) in a serological survey using IFAT in wild canids in South Carolina found that two out of 26 (8%) of gray foxes were positive for *T. cruzi* antibodies but the two coyotes tested were negative. In another paper, Rosypal et al. (2010) reported *T. cruzi* antibodies, using an immunochromatographic dipstick test (ICT), in

Table 3.3. Infection Rates, by Demonstration of the Parasite, of Two of the Most Common Wild Reservoirs of *T. cruzi* in the United States

Common Name	No. of Animals Examined	No. of Animals Positive	%	State	References
Opossum	8	8	100.0	Texas	Packchanian, 1942
	552	93	16.8	Georgia, Florida	McKeever et al., 1958
	391	63	16.1	Texas	Eads et al., 1963
	126	17	13.5	Alabama	Olsen et al., 1964
	48	18	37.5	Louisiana	Barr et al., 1991a
	12	1	8.3	North Carolina	Karsten et al., 1992
	39	6	15.3	Georgia	Pung et al., 1995
	24	16	66.6	Louisiana	Houk et al., 2010
Total	**1,200**	**222**	**18.5**		
Raccoon	608	9	1.5	Georgia, Florida	McKeever et al., 1958
	400	5	1.3	Maryland	Walton et al., 1958
	472	10	2.1	Maryland	Herman and Bruce, 1962
	35	5	14.3	Alabama	Olsen et al., 1964
	94	15	16.0	Florida, Georgia, Texas	Schaffer et al., 1978
	8	5	62.5	Oklahoma	John and Hoppe, 1986
	184	2	1.1	Florida	Telford and Forrester, 1991
	20	3	15.0	North Carolina	Karsten et al., 1992
	54	12	22.2	Georgia	Pung et al., 1995
	30	13	43.3	Georgia	Pietrzak and Pung, 1998
	3	2	66.6	Tennessee	Herwaldt et al., 2000
	83	25	30.1	Georgia	Yabsley et al., 2001
Total	**1,991**	**106**	**5.3**		

six of 49 gray foxes (11%), four captured in North Carolina and two in Virginia. None of five red foxes (*Vulpes vulpes*) presented antibodies. Brown et al. (2010) studied the seroprevalence for *T. cruzi* in 11 species of mammals from six states, also using IFAT. Besides the high number of raccoons and opossums positive from Arizona, Florida, Georgia, Missouri, and Virginia, they also found evidences of infection in striped skunks, bobcats, coyotes, and one ringtail. Houk et al. (2010), after examining by IFAT the sera of 30 opossums from southern Louisiana, found 18 (60%) of them positive. Likewise, 16 out of 24 (67%) animals of the same group yielded positive cultures for *T. cruzi*. Table 3.4 shows some details of seroprevalence rates for *T. cruzi* in potential wild reservoirs, without a direct demonstration of the parasite.

Table 3.4. Chronological Seroprevalence Rates for *T. cruzi* in Possible Local Wild Reservoirs in the United States

Common Name (Scientific Name)	Number Examined	Number Positive	%	Method	State	References
Coyote (*C. latrans*)	156	20	12.8	IHA	Texas	Burkholder et al., 1980
Badger (*T. taxus*)	8	2	25.0	IHA	Texas	Burkholder et al., 1980
Coyote (*C. latrans*)	134	19	14.2	IFAT	Texas	Grögl et al., 1984
Raccoon (*P. lotor*)	58	19	32.8	IFAT-ELISA	Georgia	Yabsley et al., 2001
Raccon (*P. lotor*)	181	87	48.1	IFAT	South Carolina	Yabsley and Noblet, 2002a
Armadillo (*Dasypus novemcinctus*)	413	16	3.9	IHA	Louisiana	Paige et al., 2002
Raccon (*P. lotor*)	464	154	33.2	IFAT	Virginia	Hancock et al., 2005
Gray Fox (*Urocyon cinereoargenteus*)	26	2	8.0	IFAT	South Carolina	Rosypal et al., 2006
Gray fox (*U. cinereoargenteus*)	49	6	12.0	ICT	North Carolina, Virginia	Rosypal et al., 2010
Coyote (*C. latrans*)	49	2	4.1	IFAT	Georgia, Virginia	Brown et al., 2010
Bobcat (*Felis rufus*)	62	2	3.2	IFAT	Georgia	Brown et al., 2010
Striped skunk (*Mephitis mephitis*)	37	4	10.8	IFAT	Arizona, Georgia	Brown et al., 2010
Raccoon (*P. lotor*)	693	280	40.4	IFAT	Arizona, Florida, Georgia, Missouri	Brown et al., 2010
Opossum (*D. virginiana*)	454	133	29.3	IFAT	Florida, Georgia, Virginia	Brown et al., 2010
Opossum (*D. virginiana*)	30	18	60.0	IFAT	Louisiana	Houk et al., 2010

Note: Brown et al. (2010) also found a single specimen of ringtail (*Bassariscus astutus*) serologically positive.

It is worth reporting here the finding of the natural infection of imported monkeys, which were most probably infected within the United States. The first case, which was fatal, was a gibbon (*Hylobates pileatus*) from Malaysia that presented inflammatory cellular infiltration and amastigotes in the myocardium. The fact that the monkey was at the Delta Regional Primate Research Center at Covington, Louisiana, led the authors to suggest the possibility of an infection via an insect vector (Seibold and Wolf, 1970). Another case occurred in an infant rhesus monkey (*Macaca mulatta*), which, after being immunosuppressed, was inoculated with the blood of another rhesus with myelogenous leukemia and which, as later demonstrated, was also infected with *T. cruzi*. The latter monkey was in Austin, Texas, for 6 years and it is unclear whether it became infected there or somewhere else in the United States (Cicmanec et al., 1974).

Kasa et al. (1977) make reference to a deceased adult female rhesus monkey that had been maintained in an outdoor primate colony in Southern Texas and showed chagasic myocarditis with multifocal pseudo-cysts. Another 20 monkeys of the same colony were also seropositive for *T. cruzi*. Several triatomines were collected from areas near the colony (Brooks Air Force Base, San Antonio, Texas) along with reservoir animals, which were common around the facility.

Of particular interest is the report of *T. cruzi* in a Colombian squirrel monkey (*Saimiri sciureus*) and her male offspring, which tested positive by microscopy, hemoculture, and xenodiagnosis while housed at the Delta Primate Center in Louisiana (Eberhard and D'Alessandro, 1982). Because the baby was raised indoors where exposure to vectors was unlikely, this is thought to represent the first report of congenital transmission in a non-human primate in the United States. A pig-tailed macaque was also identified to be positive by hemoculture, PCR, and serology (Schielke et al., 2002). Although the monkey originated in the indoor housing unit at the Washington National Primate Research Center (NPRC), it was thought to have acquired the parasite after transfer to the Tulane NPRC.

On another occasion, a 4-month-old colony baboon (*Papio cynocephalus*) died with severe diffuse myocarditis and numerous intracellular *T. cruzi* amastigotes. This was at the Southwest Foundation for Biomedical Research, also in San Antonio, Texas, where lights near cages attracted triatomines at night (Gleiser et al., 1986).

Williams et al. (2009) added three more baboons from the same place, which also died of congestive heart failure with multifocal or diffuse myocarditis, all of them showing amastigotes of *T. cruzi* in the myocardial fibers. The authors mentioned that, up to that date, 182 baboons had tested seropositive for *T. cruzi*, representing 2–3% of the entire colony.

An adult male Celebes black macaque (*Macaca nigra*) acquired from a zoo in Texas and taken to the Primate Research Center in Oregon died of chagasic encephalitis. The monkey presented at postmortem with focal areas of myocarditis and numerous amastigote forms in sections of the brain. The diagnosis had been previously established by the finding of trypanosomes in the spinal fluid of the animal, which showed signs of depression. The macaque was probably in a chronic phase of the disease when it arrived in Oregon, and the administration of corticosteroids probably triggered the clinical symptoms (Olson et al., 1986).

Pung et al. (1998) made reference to infection of Old World primates released in St. Catherines Island, Georgia. Seven out of 11 lion-tailed macaques (*Macaca silenus*) and one of 19 ring-tailed lemurs (*Lemur catta*) were found to be infected with *T. cruzi* of the same genotype as that circulating in local raccoons. *T. sanguisuga* has been found on the island, and the authors observed a macaque catching and chewing one of these bugs, which suggests possible oral transmission in these cases. Pung et al. (1998) concluded that "our findings and those of others indicate that primates and other mammals translocated to the southern part of the United States may become infected with indigenous strains of *T. cruzi*."

A survey by Hall et al. (2007) in St. Catherines Island in three species of lemurs (*Lemur catta*, *Eulemur macaco flavifrons*, and *Varecia variegata variegata*) showed a 6.5% prevalence by hemoculture only in *L. catta*, and 51.2, 20, and 75% seropositivity (ELISA test) for the three species, respectively, for a total of 50% prevalence. Molecular characterization of three *T. cruzi* isolates indicated that they belonged to Group IIa, the same group identified in raccoons from the Island. A few specimens of *T. sanguisuga* were captured but none were infected.

Bommineni et al. (2009) described a fatal acute case of Chagas disease in a 23-year-old captive chimpanzee at the Southwest NPRC in San Antonio, Texas. At necropsy, lesions were consistent with a "mild congestive heart failure" and the animal showed multifocal necrosis with amastigote nests in the myocardium. *T. cruzi* was confirmed by a PCR test and immunohistochemistry.

Nearly 2% (35 of 2,074) of the primates from the Tulane NPRC (formerly Delta Regional Primate Center) demonstrated antibodies to *T. cruzi*. Infected species included two macaque species (*M. mulatta* and *Macaca nemestrina*), a baboon (*Papio anubis*), and a gibbon (*Hylobates lar*). Because all but nine of these animals were born and raised in Louisiana, it is clear there is local transmission (Dorn et al., unpublished data).

3.2 DOGS AND OTHER DOMESTIC ANIMALS

Dogs are the most common naturally infected domestic animal in several areas of the United States. The first well-documented report of infected dogs was that of Williams et al. (1977), who reported nine acute fatal cases in Texas. All of the dogs were young (only two were older than 8 months) and all showed clinical manifestations. Amastigotes were found in myocardial fibers of the animals, which presented different degrees of diffuse granulomatous myocarditis. More than 50 specimens of *T. lecticularia* were found in a single doghouse, some of them infected, and a strain of *T. cruzi* was isolated in culture from one of the dogs.

Nissen et al. (1977) also reported a fatal case in a South Carolina puppy. Tippit (1978), based on the Texas cases, reviewed some of the facts related to canine acute trypanosomiasis and urged veterinarians to familiarize themselves with this clinical syndrome.

Snider et al. (1980) reported the finding of another lethal case, this time in a 7-month-old Labrador retriever from New Orleans, Louisiana. Two dead females of *T. sanguisuga* were found in the doghouse and a live male was found in a closet of the owner's residence. Another acute case was found in Oklahoma in a 13-year-old female Labrador retriever that showed weakness, fever, and edemas. Parasites were found in the peripheral blood and amastigotes were found in the cardiac muscle after euthanizing the animal. Four more dogs from different parts of Oklahoma were found to be serologically positive (Fox et al., 1986).

In a series of papers, Barr and collaborators performed detailed studies on natural and experimental canine trypanosomiasis at the School of Veterinary Medicine at Louisiana State University. The first animal studied was a 12-year-old spayed female Labrador retriever with fever, dyspnea, stridor, retching, arrhythmia, and laryngeal paralysis and with *T. cruzi* in the peripheral blood. The dead animal showed myocardial degeneration with fibrosis and lesions in the liver and skeletal muscle, but amastigotes were not detected (Barr et al. 1986). Barr et al. (1989) also reported a case of two adult hunting dogs from Louisiana with signs typical of chronic passive congestion attributable to Chagas disease. Both had cardiomegaly, first-degree heart block, and ECG abnormalities consistent with right bundle branch block (RBBB). In both animals, similar histopathological changes were found; the myocardial fibers were separated by interstitial edema, and multifocal fibrosis was evident. In one of them, intracellular amastigotes were observed.

Barr et al. (1995) described *T. cruzi* infection in eight of nine littermates born to an infected but clinically asymptomatic Walker hound from Augusta County, Virginia. Parasites were seen in blood smears from all but one pup. Necropsies revealed amastigotes in the cardiac fibers in three of four pups and also in the nervous system. Barr et al. (1995) inferred that this type of infection is more prevalent than previously thought and emphasized the fact that "North American isolates of *T. cruzi* may be as pathogenic to human beings as are South American isolates."

Berger et al. (1991) mentioned the occurrence of neurological dysfunction in dogs infected with *T. cruzi* and reported a case of a 13-month-old Doberman pinscher from Texas with progressive paraparesis, severe granulomatosis myocarditis, and meningoencephalitis at necropsy, with intracellular clusters of amastigotes, including in sections of the spinal cord.

Woods et al. (2000) made reference to a 4-month-old English Mastiff, examined at the Oklahoma State University Veterinary School, with weight loss, lymphadenopathy, and pyrexia, which revealed trypomastigotes in the lymph node aspirates. *T. cruzi* was also cultured from the same material, and an indirect immunofluorescent antibody test showed a significant positive titer. Another similar case was reported more recently in an 8-month English Mastiff from Texas, with subcutaneous edema, lymphadenopathy, and loss of weight. A lymph node aspirate revealed amastigotes of *T. cruzi*, which were also confirmed by culture, serology, and a PCR test (Nabity ct al., 2006).

In a retrospective study based on clinical histories from the Texas Veterinary Medical Diagnostic Laboratory, Meurs et al. (1998) studied the chronic stage of the disease and pointed out that the main clinical signs are exercise intolerance, lethargy, ascites, tachycardia, and inappetence. ECG abnormalities were detected in 10 of 11 dogs, consisting of arrhythmias and conduction disturbances, and the most common was RBBB, paralleling that reported in humans with chronic Chagas disease. Echocardiograms also detected abnormalities in all dogs examined.

Serological surveys have also been performed on dogs. Burkholder et al. (1980), using the IHA test, examined 136 stray dogs in Texas and found 12 reactive (8.8%). Tomlinson et al. (1981) analyzed the sera of 365 dogs from Georgia and other southeastern states by complement fixation test and found seven positive animals with no signs of the disease. Vakalis et al. (1983) performed a direct agglutination test (DAT) and an IHA on 174 dogs from the West Bank area of New Orleans, Louisiana, and found two positive animals. One of them was asymptomatic and the other had ataxia and a cardiovascular problem. Navin et al. (1985) made reference to the finding of six serologically positive dogs from the area of Lake Don Pedro, California, and Herwaldt et al. (2000) reported finding one positive dog, also by serology, in Tennessee. Barr et al. (1991d) made reference to a 4.7% seropositivity rate in a group of 85 roaming dogs from rural Louisiana that had elevated exposure to wild mammals; other groups, such as 103 housed rural and 176 roaming urban dogs, showed lower rates of 2 and 2.3%, respectively. The authors also reported two serologically positive dogs out of 52 examined from a location in Virginia, where they found eight infected littermates born to an infected Walker hound (Barr et al., 1995). Bradley et al. (2000), using RIPA technique, found 11 seropositive dogs out of 304 examined (3.6%) in three counties of eastern Oklahoma. They isolated the parasite from one animal and identified it as *T. cruzi* by PCR testing. The authors also made reference to three previously infected dogs from the same area. Beard et al. (2003) reported three pet dogs that died from Chagas myocardiopathy in San Benito, Texas. Serological tests (IIF) of seven dogs from two houses, one of them where the dogs had died, revealed four to be infected; moreover, of 375 stray dogs from Cameron county, 28 (7.5%) were seropositive. Shadomy et al. (2004) searched for *T. cruzi* antibodies in 356 domestic dogs from Harris County, Texas, and surrounding areas by combining an ELISA test with flow cytometry as a confirmatory technique and found an overall prevalence of 2.6%.

In a serological survey for visceral leishmaniasis in foxhound dogs, Duprey et al. (2006) found that 86 out of 413 animals (21%), originating from 13 states, were positive for *T. cruzi* antibodies, as revealed by a radioimmunoprecipitation assay (RIPA).

Kjos et al. (2008) have reviewed the situation of canine Chagas disease in the United States and have presented an extensive report based on 537 serologically (ELISA and IIF) and histopathologically confirmed cases, originating in 48 Texas counties, and corresponding to a period of about 15 years. Acute cases occurred in 42% of necropsied animals, over half of them less than a year old. Myocarditis was frequent (97.9%) in this group, and amastigotes were found in 81.7% of the cases. Dogs from both urban and rural areas were affected, although illness was more common in sporting and working breeds. Cardiac dysfunction was a major problem among several other clinical observations.

Nieto et al. (2009) reported high levels of seropositivity (16 of 31 dogs; 51.6%) by IFAT in three kennels in Louisiana housing hunting dogs, Labrador Retrievers, and Beagles. *T. sanguisuga* was also found in one kennel. In a survey of dogs from local veterinary practices, by using IFAT, 11 of 91 (12%) of the dogs contained *T. cruzi* antibodies for a total of 27 animals out of 122 (22.1% positive). The authors also compared IFAT with two rapid immunochromatographic assays, finding them similar in sensitivity and specificity and recommending the rapid tests to veterinarians for the diagnosis of Chagas disease in dogs.

In conclusion, dogs infected with *T. cruzi* have been found in at least eight states (in California, Georgia, and Tennessee only by serology), and a more careful search will probably show that they are commonly infected in several other areas of the country. Dogs can easily become infected when they catch bugs with their mouths and chew them (Williams et al., 1977; Wood and Wood, 1964a; Zeledón, 1974). Hunting dogs probably can also become infected through exposure to infected wild reservoirs. Some other domestic animals have been found serologically to be infected with *T. cruzi*. Burkholder et al. (1980) reported the finding of antibodies in 14 out of 43 (32.6%) cows (*Bos taurus*) and in four out of 30 sheep (*Ovis aries*) in Texas, by using the IHA test.

CHAPTER 4

The Parasite

4.1 EXPERIMENTAL INFECTIONS IN ANIMALS

One mechanism used to learn more about the biological characteristics of the parasite is to inoculate laboratory, domestic, and/or wild animals with isolates obtained from different sources. Numerous animals have been experimentally infected with *T. cruzi* strains isolated in the United States. In this section, we summarize the main experiments, without being exhaustive, showing that some isolates produce mild infections whereas others can lead to severe pathological lesions and even to death, in the same manner as occurs with Central and South American strains, as indicated in the literature.

Kofoid and Donat (1933a) were the first to successfully inoculate albino rats, the dusky-footed rat (*N. f. annectans*), and an opossum (*D. virginiana*), either with *T. protracta* feces, which were naturally associated with the wood rats, or with infected blood from an albino rat. These authors were able to demonstrate the amastigote forms of the parasite in the tissues of the laboratory rat.

By using the same California strain, Wood (1934a) infected a series of animals including albino mice, dogs, opossums, rhesus monkeys (*Macaca mulatta*), San Diego wood rats, Portola wood rats, and white-footed mice (*Peromyscus* spp.). At least one of each of these animals became infected, and in all cases the infection was mild. The authors were unable to infect rabbits, guinea pigs, kittens, and one desert antelope ground squirrel.

Packchanian (1939) injected several animals with the feces of infected *T. gerstaeckeri* from Texas. Of 44 animals inoculated, 34 became infected, including laboratory mice, two species of *Peromyscus*, guinea pigs, and rhesus monkeys. In all animals, the parasitemia was low, and amastigotes were found in the tissues of some of them. The same author was able to infect these animals with a strain isolated from *T. lecticularia* from Texas and also infected mice and guinea pigs with a strain of *T. cruzi* obtained from experimentally infected *T. sanguisuga* from Florida (Packchanian, 1940b). In another experiment, two rhesus monkeys infected with an isolate from a wood rat (*N. m. micropus*) showed amastigotes in some tissues (Packchanian, 1942).

Davis (1943) infected several rhesus monkeys from Texas and California by dropping the fecal material of infected bugs (*T. gerstaeckeri* and *T. protracta*) into one eye. Parasites were observed in the blood as early as 14 days and up to 58 days after inoculation. The animals had fever, and three of them presented a typical bipalpebral edema in the eye even though the preauricular or cervical lymph nodes were not palpable. Postmortem histopathological studies revealed mild diffuse myocarditis with amastigotes in the heart muscle. Human strains from Panama and Venezuela produced the same clinical picture in some other infected monkeys.

Diamond and Rubin (1956) inoculated six pigs, four lambs, and two goats, all 1 day old, with the Patuxent raccoon isolate of *T. cruzi*. In sheep and goats, a mild- and short-term parasitemia was observed, and parasites were recovered in cultures; only the pigs yielded a positive culture. No symptoms were observed, but typical amastigotes were found in the heart muscle of a pig and of a goat. In another paper, the authors give more details of the experiment and add calves, which responded in a similar way to the other farm animals (Diamond and Rubin, 1958).

Walton et al. (1958) were able to infect several animals, including raccoons, with the same raccoon strain from the Patuxent Research Refuge of Maryland. The infection was mild in all animals, which included laboratory mice and rats, opossums, and monkeys (*Macaca irus*).

Goble (1958) studied the infectivity and pathogenicity of five *T. cruzi* isolates (Corpus Christi and Texas strains from two indigenous human cases and one isolate from a raccoon, one from a human case from Brazil, and one from *T. infestans* from Chile) by inoculating 10-week-old dogs. The Brazilian isolate produced the highest parasitemia and mortality (80%), whereas the Houston isolate yielded low to no mortality. On the other hand, the Corpus Christi isolate produced a mortality of 35%, similar to the Chilean isolate (Tulahuen), and the raccoon (Patuxent) isolate failed to kill any animal. In an extension of these experiments, the dogs infected with the avirulent Houston strain were subsequently challenged with the more virulent Corpus Christi and Brazil strains and were protected. The same was observed in dogs, which survived challenge with Corpus Christi and Brazilian strains (Goble, 1961).

In a series of papers, Barr and collaborators reported on pathological findings observed in experimental infections of dogs with North American strains of *T. cruzi*. In the first report (Barr et al., 1991b), 19 pure-bred Beagle dogs between 4 and 47 weeks old, divided into three groups and inoculated with *T. cruzi* isolates from opossum, armadillo, and dog, respectively, yielded the following results. Dogs of the first group developed severe acute disease and some died; dogs of the second group also had acute disease but survived and entered an early chronic phase with a positive serology; and dogs of the third group developed neither acute nor symptomatic chronic disease. The disease was more severe in the younger dogs (4–5 weeks) and in dogs that developed chronic infection; signs were associated with gradual loss of cardiac function. In the third group of dogs inoculated with a less virulent or avirulent canine-derived strain, the only clinical sign was lymphoadenopathy. Signs of acute myocarditis in some of the dogs were similar to those of people, and the authors concluded that there was an agreement of their results with those of experimental infections of dogs in South America.

In another report (Barr et al., 1991e), the authors studied the humoral and cellular immune response of dogs to a nonpathogenic canine *T. cruzi* isolate and to a pathogenic opossum-derived strain, during a period of 8 months. Antibodies detected by ELISA were present by day 26 and peaked by day 175, with no marked difference in the two groups of dogs; the blastogenic responses of peripheral blood mononuclear cells were also similar.

Barr et al. (1991c) also studied the pathological changes that occurred in 23 Beagles inoculated with the same three *T. cruzi* isolates. The canine strain induced minor histological changes as expected, while dogs from the other groups, which survived the acute phase, developed chronic pathological changes similar to those found in dogs with naturally acquired infection and similar to lesions described in chronic human Chagas disease. These authors thoroughly describe the pathological findings in dogs with both the acute phase and the chronic phase of the disease.

Finally, Barr et al. (1992) observed the ECG and echocardiographic changes in the same dogs during or after the acute phase. Although those infected with the dog isolate did not develop cardiac abnormalities, the

ones inoculated with the raccoon or opossum strains showed ECG alterations such as increases in P-R intervals, atrioventricular blocks, depression in R wave amplitude, and shifts in mean electrical axis during the
acute myocarditis period. In the cases that entered into an early chronic
phase, there was a progression of ECG changes. Ventricular-based
arrhythmias and premature multifocal ventricular contractions started
in some dogs after 60 and 170 postinoculation days. ECG abnormalities
were concomitant with loss of left ventricular function as revealed by
echocardiography, with a mean ejection fraction and fractional shorten-
ing that decreased 63 and 52%, respectively, in relation to control values.

Numerous authors have infected laboratory mice with different U.S.
isolates of *T. cruzi* mainly for comparative purposes. In the following
paragraphs, we summarize some of these experiments.

Wood (1934b) described the presence of broad and slender forms of
the parasite in the peripheral blood of mouse. This morphological characteristic was first observed by Chagas himself, and both forms may be
present in different proportions in *T. cruzi* strains. The possible biological significance of this polymorphism has been critically reviewed by
Brener (1973).

Kofoid et al. (1935) were able to reproduce the vertebrate developmental stages of the parasite in mouse and rat embryonic heart tissue culture, which was infected with a Californian wood rat isolate. They also
used the above heart tissue culture system to test the action of arsenical
drugs on the intracellular form of the parasite (Kofoid et al., 1937).

Wood (1941b) observed that New Mexico and Arizona strains were
able to produce higher parasitemias in mice than a California strain;
nevertheless, an isolate from Eaton Canyon, California, was able to kill
the mice, and one mouse showed nervous symptoms indicating a neuro-
tropism by this strain.

Lesser and Lukerman (1957) were able to infect Swiss Albino mice
with the Corpus Christi human strain and were able to find amastigotes
in the muscle of the stomach, esophagus, and small intestine, as well as
in the heart. Norman et al. (1959) inoculated mice with five isolates from
opossum, skunk, and raccoon, observing a low parasitemia (an opossum
strain did not infect the mice). Amastigotes were observed in the heart,
and variations within a single strain were also observed.

In their review article, Kagan et al. (1966) summarized some experiments in mice with North American strains, including their own work. They concluded that the strains could be divided into three main groups. In group I, they included the moderately pathogenic strains, such as "human Corpus Christi," which produced parasitemias in 87% of the mice with 63% mortality. In group II, they placed the slightly virulent strains (opossum) with parasitemias in 50% of the mice and less than 10% mortality. In group III, they included the strains with very low virulence (raccoon, skunk, and opossum), which produced parasitemias in less than 20% of the mice and less than 10% mortality. The authors also remarked that the strains have different tissue tropisms and that nonpathogenic strains can protect against new challenges with pathogenic ones.

While infecting DF1 mice with three Louisiana strains from dog, armadillo, and opossum, Barr et al. (1990a) confirmed some heterogeneity between them. Armadillo and opossum isolates were similar and produced more pathological alterations in tissues than the dog isolate.

4.2 MOLECULAR CHARACTERIZATION OF ISOLATES

In comparison with work done in Latin America on the molecular characterization of isolates from different origins, rather few contributions are available with U.S. strains. The strain isolated from the first indigenous California case of Chagas disease was examined by isoenzyme patterns, and it was observed that it corresponded to zymodeme I even though two enzymes showed a different pattern (Navin et al., 1985).

Beard et al. (1988) characterized the parasite that they isolated in Florida from *T. sanguisuga*, and the isoenzyme profile showed that it belonged to the zymodeme I group.

Barr et al. (1990b) compared the three strains mentioned above, from a dog, an armadillo, and an opossum, in axenic and tissue cultures, with respect to protein profiles and isoenzyme pattern. There was a marked difference between the dog and the two wild animal isolates in the kinetics of trypomastigote–cell adherence and internalization rate, with an evident slower rate in the former isolate. Both the armadillo and the opossum strains grouped into zymodeme I, but the dog isolate pattern did not correspond to the reference stocks.

Clark and Pung (1994) proposed the term "ribodeme" to describe populations of a species that share the same riboprint pattern. They identified as ribodeme I the isolates from raccoon and *T. sanguisuga*, together with three Brazilian human isolates, and as ribodeme II the opossum isolate. Another human isolate from Brazil was classified as ribodeme III. Pung et al. (1995) used the same molecular technique to confirm *T. cruzi* taxon isolated from wild animals or from triatomine origin.

Barr et al. (1995), by using PCR assays, also made a molecular characterization of an isolate from a dog, confirming it as *T. cruzi*. Pung et al. (1998) observed a different rDNA polymorphism pattern and a distinct amplification product size among raccoon and nonhuman primate isolates, from St. Catherines Island in Georgia, and opossum isolates.

Barnabé et al. (2001) compared patterns generated independently by isoenzyme and RAPD analysis to evaluate phylogenetic divergence among 30 U.S.-derived *T. cruzi* stocks isolated primarily from wild mammals and triatomine vectors. Both methods demonstrated a high degree of genetic diversity among the stocks, which were resolved into two primary lineages, corresponding to the previously described zymodemes I and III. Additionally, the authors observed a high degree of correlation in the results determined by the two approaches. From the results, they hypothesized that U.S. *T. cruzi* stocks were not imported at a historical time but rather were indigenous to native fauna of the region.

Yabsley and Noblet (2002b) characterized by biological and molecular methods (isoenzyme analysis, RAPD-PCR, and amplification of the nontranscribed region of the mini-exon gene) a low virulent strain from a raccoon, comparing it with a Brazilian virulent strain. The raccoon strain behaved as *T. cruzi* group II (Lineage 1). The authors were also able to detect DNA of *T. cruzi* in mice tissues by PCR.

Roelling et al. (2008) analyzed 107 U.S. isolates of *T. cruzi* from different origins (captive wildlife, domestic animals, triatomines, and humans) and concluded that only two genotypes were involved in these various hosts. Isolates from Virginia opossum, triatomines, humans, and rhesus macaques were characterized as type I and those from one non-human primate, raccoons, lemurs, skunks, and domestic dogs were characterized as type IIa. The authors concluded that the two main phylogenetic clusters found confirmed previous findings (Barnabé et al., 2001) and that opossums primarily maintain infections with *T. cruzi* I whereas raccoons are usually infected with type IIa. These findings were reinforced by Roelling et al. (2009), after experimental infection of small groups of raccoons and opossums with identified isolates belonging to types I, IIa, and IIb (Brazilian strain). Parasitemia was only detected in opossums inoculated with *T. cruzi* I or with both types together; conversely, tissue forms of Tc IIa or Tc IIb were not even demonstrated by PCR in these animals and cultures were negative. On the contrary, raccoons were more easily infected with *T. cruzi* type IIa. The new intraspecific nomenclature launched at the Second Satellite Meeting in Brazil (Zingales et al., 2009) divided *T. cruzi* into six distinct DRUs (discrete typing units) and classified one strain from *D. marsupialis* of Georgia as *T. cruzi* I and another strain, also from Georgia from *P. lotor*, as *T. cruzi* IV. A third strain from a domestic dog from Oklahoma was also considered to be *T. cruzi* IV.

Hwang et al. (2010), using ribosomal RNA genes, found two genotypes of *T. cruzi* isolates from *T. protracta* captured in southern California, and these were closely related to TcII and TcVI. Cura et al. (2010) used the SL-IR gene to identify genotypes TcIa of *T. cruzi* infecting *T. gerstaeckeri* from Texas and *D. virginiana* from Florida. New systematic work is necessary to clarify the meaning of the different genotypes already identified, according to the new genetic concepts of the different stocks.

CHAPTER 5

Prevalence of Chagas Disease in Human Beings

5.1 INDIGENOUS CASES

Although the agent and the vector of Chagas disease were reported to exist in the United States just 7 years after Carlos Chagas discovered the new trypanosomiasis in Brazil, it was not until almost 40 years later that an indigenous case was demonstrated. The finding of other possible vectors, in addition to the natural infection of several wild mammals with the parasite, may have lead some scientists in later decades to believe that the strains of the parasite that were circulating in the United States were not virulent enough to infect humans (Packchanian, 1943). Other hypotheses that attempted to explain the apparent absence of infection were the rather sporadic contact between humans and insect, the low density of bugs in human dwellings, better home construction, the inefficiency of the local bugs in transmitting the parasite, and the fact that physicians considered Chagas disease to be a remote tropical illness and were unaware of its symptoms (Burkholder et al., 1980; Farrar et al., 1963; Martins, 1968; Navin et al., 1985; Tonn, 1985; Woody and Woody, 1961; Yaeger, 1959).

In December 1940, a 24-year-old man was inoculated in his left eye with material obtained from an infected bug (*T. lecticularia*) in Texas. Fever began 2 weeks after exposure, the left eyelids became swollen and edematous, and trypanosomes became evident in peripheral blood 21 days after the infection. Cultures yielded positive results from 21 to 84 days after inoculation, and laboratory animals were infected with the patient's blood. In September 1942 (21 months later), the patient was seen again and appeared to be normal. Although this experiment must be considered to be unethical, it was the first demonstration "that the Texas strain of *T. cruzi* is capable of infecting man with a disease clinically identical with that known as Chagas disease or South American trypanosomiasis" (Packchanian, 1943).

Packchanian (1947) stated that "the epidemiologic factors necessary to its occurrence in human beings have been shown repeatedly to be

An Appraisal of the Status of Chagas Disease in the United States. DOI: 10.1016/B978-0-12-397268-2.00005-5

present in numerous sections of Texas and the Southwest" and added that "It is my firm opinion that Chagas' disease exists in man in Texas" but he claimed that physicians were not aware of this possibility and were not familiar with the clinical symptoms.

Dias (1951) reviewed the apparent absence of the disease during the first half of the 20th century in the United States and gathered together the opinions of some American scientists, who agreed that the first auto-chthonous case could be detected at any time. This Brazilian author, accompanied by the cardiologist Francisco Laranja, visited the School of Medicine of the University of Texas, at Galveston, in 1946, and observed the records showing altered ECGs provided by Dr. G. Herrmann, which suggested Chagas myocardiopathy. A few altered ECGs were selected and given to Dr. Packchanian, from the same school, who later demon-strated that a subset of these patients were serologically positive for *T. cruzi.*

In 1955, a 10-month-old female child from the vicinity of Corpus Christi, Texas, became the first diagnosed case of indigenous Chagas disease in the United States. The child showed fever, edema of the face, posterior auricular adenopathy, and lymphocytosis. Leukemia was suspected, but trypanosomes were observed while examining a blood smear. The parasite was isolated in culture, and it was con-firmed that family members had been bitten by triatomine bugs at the infant's home. Some of the bugs found in the home were infected, and opossums were known to be common in the vicinity (Woody and Woody, 1955, 1964).

The second case was discovered just a few months latter, in November 1955, in a 6-month-old male. The infant, originally from Bryan County, Texas, became ill when he was 2–3 weeks old and was admitted to the hospital in Houston with a diagnosis of salmonellosis. He received four blood transfusions at the hospital and at month 5; after an obstructive hydrocephalus, a laboratory technician observed trypanosomes in the cerebrospinal fluid, which were successfully cultured (Anonymous, 1955, 1956; Woody and Woody, 1964). In this case, no triatomine bugs were found in the house or vicinity where the child lived, suggesting that the child was infected through a blood transfusion.

The third indigenous case of Chagas disease was discovered in Cali-fornia in a 56-year-old woman from Lake Don Pedro, 120 miles east of

San Francisco. She was admitted to the hospital after 16 days of fever, and trypanosomes were observed in a thin peripheral blood smear. The parasite was isolated in culture, and mice were infected with the strain. The patient, who had never had a blood transfusion and had never traveled to an endemic area, was treated successfully with nifurtimox for 120 days, and CF serological tests became negative after treatment (Schiffler et al., 1984). Navin et al. (1985) added some epidemiological information to this case. Six dogs from the area yielded positive serology, and *T. cruzi* was isolated from two ground squirrels caught a few miles from the patient's house. One *T. protracta* was found in the patient's bathroom, and two others were found in neighboring houses. *T. protracta* specimens were also found in wood rat dens in the area, and some were infected. Finally, six residents of Lake Don Pedro gave a positive CF test out of 241 people examined.

The fourth case of indigenous Chagas disease was reported in a 7-month-old boy from South Texas (Ochs et al., 1996). The child entered the hospital in 1983 with fever, liver and spleen enlargement, and myocarditis, but Chagas disease was not suspected during the 3 days that preceded the child's death. A year later, new slides of cardiac tissue revealed amastigotes of *T. cruzi*, and 7 years later this was confirmed in cardiac tissue by PCR. Transfusion-associated and congenital transmissions were ruled out in this case even though no bugs were found in the patient's house, although typical habitats for the insect were common in the surroundings.

Another case occurred in Tennessee in 1998 in an 18-month-old boy who was diagnosed only by PCR. The child was intermittently febrile and showed multiple insect bites on his legs. An adult female *T. sanguisuga* was found by the child's mother in his crib and sent to a local university for identification. It was demonstrated later at the CDC in Atlanta that the insect was infected with *T. cruzi*. Several direct blood examinations and hemocultures from the child yielded negative results, as did conventional serological tests (IIF, ELISA, and latex agglutination) but the PCR positive reaction prompted the physicians to start treatment with benznidazole (Roche), and the PCR became negative about 5 months later. Serological tests in 19 family members and neighbors were negative but one of the family's two dogs was positive. Two out of three raccoons from the area yielded a positive culture. A single immature-stage insect was found in a wood pile on a neighbor's farm, and one *T. sanguisuga* female was found by the family in their basement and another on the front porch (Herwaldt et al., 2000).

The latest and most recent case took place in rural New Orleans in a 74-year-old woman bothered by insect bites. Trypanosomes were cultured from the patient 4 months later. Serology of the patient was positive (Loyola University New Orleans and CDC), and she was and remains asymptomatic. Approximately half of the *T. sanguisuga* (18 adult specimens) found in and around the house were shown to be *T. cruzi*-positive by PCR (Dorn et al., 2007).

The main characteristics of the six indigenous cases found in the country to date are presented in Table 5.1.

An extensive literature review, aiming to substantiate the assertion that Chagas disease is endemic to Texas, has been published by Hanford et al. (2007). The authors concluded that the disease represents a greater threat as an emerging disease than previously thought and that there is a need for research leading to a better understanding of its prevalence, transmission, spread, and severity in Texas and other areas of the country.

On the basis of the distribution of the autochthonous human cases in the United States, Lambert et al. (2008), using geographical information system (GIS) analysis, depicted the higher risk areas for vectorial transmission, with projections to the year 2030, following predicted climate changes. They believe that there will be increasing potential for the emergence of Chagas disease in the country, and, after completing a physician's survey, claimed that "Chagas disease is not always considered as a possible diagnosis in the area defined to be at increased risk in the United States."

Sarkar et al. (2010) extended the distribution of vector species to 10 new counties of Texas. By constructing species distribution models based on available and new information, they concluded that the disease is endemic in some sites in Texas. They also recommended making Chagas disease a reportable disease in Texas; screening all blood samples donated from persons from high-risk countries; performing serological surveys in humans and dogs; and creating a Mexican–U.S. new initiative to combat Chagas disease.

Table 5.1. Autochthonous Chagas Disease Cases in the United States

Case No.	Age	Sex	Origin	Symptoms	Diagnostic Method	Serology	Vectors	Treatment	References
1	10 months	F	Corpus Christi, Texas	Fever, face edema, adenitis	Blood smear, culture	Positive (CF)	T. gerstaeckeri close to the house	None	Woody and Woody, 1955; Woody et al., 1965
2	6 months	M	Bryan, Texas	Fever, obstructive hydrocephalus	Fresh cerebrospinal fluid and culture	Not done	None	None	Anonymous, 1955, 1956
3	56 years	F	Lake Don Pedro, California	Fever	Blood smear, culture	Positive (CF)	T. protracta in the house	Nifurtimox	Navin et al., 1985; Schiffler et al., 1984
4	7 months	M	South Texas	Fever, myocarditis	Histopathology and PCR (post-mortem)	Not done	None	None	Ochs et al., 1996
5	18 months	M	Rutherford County, Tennessee	Fever	PCR	Negative (PCR positive)	T. sanguisuga in the house	Benznidazole	Herwaldt et al., 2000
6	74 years	F	New Orleans, Louisiana	Asymptomatic	Culture	Positive (IFA, dipstick)	T. sanguisuga in the house	None	Dorn et al., 2007

5.2 SEROLOGICAL PREVALENCE IN HUMANS

The first attempt to serologically demonstrate infection by *T. cruzi* in the United States was that by Davis and Sullivan (1946). They examined a total of 1,909 sera samples from different counties in Texas by the CF test; of these samples, 568 were mainly from students of Mexican origin. Just one 8-year-old boy from Uvalde County yielded a positive reaction, and the authors concluded that "On the basis of this evidence it appears that American trypanosomiasis, if present at all, is extremely rare in Texas."

Woody et al. (1961) carried out a survey in the vicinity of Corpus Christi using Freitas CF test. They examined 500 individuals (466 were children), mainly of Latin American origin. Seven children tested positive, along with two adults from their families. All nine positive cases (1.8%) had been bitten by *T. gerstaeckeri*, and infected insects of this species were found in two of the houses of the positive patients. Two children had a history of "systemic illness," another one of a Romaña's sign, and of the two adults one showed incomplete right bundle branch block, as revealed by the ECG. However, the agent was not directly demonstrated in any of the patients.

Farrar et al. (1963) also did a serological survey using the CF test in three groups of patients: 1,474 sera from the wards and clinics of Grady Memorial Hospital (Atlanta), 449 sera from the State Health Department Laboratory, and 28 specimens from patients in the Cardiac Clinic at the same hospital, all with the diagnosis of "diffuse myocardial disease." Two positive reactions were obtained from each group (0.4% for the first two groups and 7.1% for the latter). One of the two positive cases with cardiac disease exhibited an abnormally wide QRS-T with left ventricular hypertrophy in the ECG, and the other one showed a left bundle branch block and had a cerebral embolism. The authors concluded that some cases of unexplained heart disease in this area may be caused by *T. cruzi*. Attempts to demonstrate the parasite in the seropositive patients were unsuccessful.

A group of 132 sera from people from Texas with a history of having been bitten by bugs and ranging in age from 10 months to 72 years were tested by Woody et al. (1965); 15 were anticomplementary and only three (2.5%) yielded positive reactions – 5.5, 42, and 72 years old, respectively. The authors mentioned that the first autochthonous case of Chagas disease from Corpus Christi still had a serologically positive reaction 10 years after the acute onset.

In another survey in a community near San Antonio, Texas, Lathrop and Ominsky (1965) had the opportunity to examine 108 sera with the CF test. Forty-eight samples belonged to people with a history of having been bitten by triatomines, and only one reaction was positive, in a 63-year-old man.

Farrar et al. (1972) tried to confirm the finding of positive serological cases in the state of Georgia, using the CF test, but failed to find any. In 3,761 unselected sera, all results were negative and 54 sera from patients with primary myocardial disease were likewise negative. These results led the authors to draw the conclusion that "In the United States this infection may affect wild animals almost exclusively."

Burkholder et al. (1980) made reference to a positive serology survey carried out in residents of the Texas Lower Rio Grande Valley. From 500 sera examined, 12 (2.4%) had significant antibody titers to *T. cruzi* by the CF test. Nevertheless, only four of these were confirmed at the CDC (0.8%). At least one of the positive cases suffered from an unexplained cardiomyopathy. The authors concluded that Chagas disease exists in the area, although at a relatively low rate.

The main results of these serological surveys have been summarized in Table 5.2.

Table 5.2. Serological Surveys for Chagas Infection in U.S. Native-Born People					
Location	No. of Persons Examined	No. of Persons Positive for *T. cruzi*	%	Type of Reaction	References
Texas	1,909	1	0.05	CF	Davis and Sullivan, 1946
Corpus Christi, Texas	500	9	1.8	CF	Woody et al., 1961
Georgia	1,474	6	0.40	CF	Farrar et al., 1963
Texas	132	3	2.27	CF	Woody et al., 1965
San Antonio, Texas	108	1	0.92	CF	Lathrop and Ominsky, 1965
Lower Rio Grande Valley, Texas	500	12	2.4	CF IHA	Burkholder et al., 1980
Lake Don Pedro, California	241	6	2.48	CF	Navin et al., 1985
Total	4,864	38	0.78		

5.3 BLOOD TRANSFUSION, AND CONGENITAL AND ORGAN TRANSPLANT TRANSMISSION

It is well-known that Chagas disease is also transmitted by blood transfusion, particularly in some areas of Latin America, where it may be transmitted at relatively high frequency (Schmuñis, 1991). This route of transmission has occurred in the United States and Canada (n = 7), with five and two published cases, respectively. Geiseler et al. (1987) reported the case of a 17-year-old resident of Watsonville, California, who died of Chagas myocarditis probably acquired through a transfusion from his father. The father had emigrated from Mexico and was subsequently shown to be serologically positive. The patient was under immunosuppression after receiving a bone marrow transplant from his sister. The autopsy revealed parasites in the myocardial cells.

In 1989, almost simultaneously, two additional cases of transfusion-transmitted *T. cruzi* were reported in North America: one from Manitoba, Canada, and the other from New York City (Grant et al., 1989; Nickerson et al., 1989). The first case involved a 21-year-old Cree Indian woman with acute lymphoblastic leukemia who was undergoing chemotherapy when numerous trypanosomes were observed on a buffy coat preparation of her blood. The patient had previously received a platelet transfusion from a person who had lived in Paraguay. The platelet donor later tested positive for Chagas disease. Upon treatment with nifurtimox, the patient improved significantly. The second case occurred in a splenectomized 11-year-old girl from the Bronx in New York City who was being treated for Hodgkin's disease. As part of her treatment, she received platelets from an asymptomatic woman who had emigrated from Bolivia. The patient demonstrated trypanosomes on a peripheral blood smear but subsequently improved following treatment with nifurtimox. The donor, upon evaluation, presented with an IIF-positive reaction for Chagas disease.

Another apparent case of transfusion-acquired Chagas disease was reported in a 59-year-old woman with metastatic colon cancer from Houston, Texas (Cimo et al., 1993). The patient was immunosuppressed due to cancer chemotherapy and received over 500 units of blood by transfusion. After investigating 40 donors, all were serologically negative, yet there was no other reasonable explanation for *T. cruzi* infection except by transfusion. The patient had demonstrable trypanosomes in her peripheral blood and bone marrow with fever, congestive heart failure, cardiac rhythm disturbances, and cardiogenic shock that ultimately proved fatal.

Two additional cases from Miami, Florida, and Providence, Rhode Island, have been reported. The first case was in a 60-year-old woman with multiple myeloma who received platelets from an infected but asymptomatic donor who had emigrated from Chile 33 years earlier. Parasites were demonstrable in the patient's blood by PCR and hemoculture before she died of complications associated with the myeloma (Leiby et al., 1999). The Rhode Island case involved a 5-year-old girl who acquired Chagas disease while under chemotherapy for a neuroblastoma (Saulnier-Sholler et al., 2006; Young et al., 2007). The implicated donor was originally from Bolivia and had emigrated to the United States 17 years earlier. In both of these cases, the implicated donor remained parasitemic and capable of transmitting infection many years after leaving their country of birth.

The second Canadian case of transfusion-transmitted *T. cruzi* also occurred in Manitoba. In this case, a 37-year-old man with prolymphocytic leukemia was confirmed to be infected with *T. cruzi* by PCR (Lane et al., 2000). A single donor from 294 tested was confirmed as seropositive for *T. cruzi*. Interestingly, similarly to the previous Canadian case, the donor was a Mennonite who donated at the same clinic as the donor involved in the previous case. The donor was born in Germany but had been raised in rural Paraguay before immigrating to Canada. In general, all seven U.S. and Canadian patients acquired the disease when they were immunosuppressed and most of them received platelets from an asymptomatic donor from an endemic area, usually a South American country. A summary with the main characteristics of these seven North American cases is presented in Table 5.3.

It remains surprising, given the significant number of seropositive blood donors identified over the past 3 years in the United States, that only five cases of transfusion transmission have been reported. Early on, Kirchhoff et al. (1987) remarked that housing quality and the absence of domiciliary bugs could explain the rarity of vectorial transmission of *T. cruzi* in the United States; nevertheless, they considered transfusion-associated transmission just as viable and, for this reason, in need of attention. The same authors performed a serological study in 205 Central Americans (10 Nicaraguans and 195 Salvadorans) living in the vicinity of Washington D.C. and found that 10 subjects showed antibodies to

Case No.	Age (years)	Sex	Donor	Origin	Condition	Diagnosis	Treatment	References
1	17	M	Mexican man	Watsonville, California	Bone marrow transplant	Autopsy (myocarditis)	None	Geisleer et al., 1987
2	11	F	Bolivian woman	Bronx, New York	Hodgkin's disease	Blood smear	Nifurtimox	Grant et al., 1989
3	21	F	Paraguayan man	Manitoba, Canada	Acute lymphoblastic leukemia	Blood smear	Nifurtimox	Nickerson et al., 1989
4	59	F	Unknown origin	Houston, Texas	Cancer	Blood smear Bone marrow	None	Cimo et al., 1993
5	60	F	Chilean woman	Miami, Florida	Multiple myeloma	Hemoculture PCR	None	Leiby et al., 1999
6	37	M	Paraguayan-raised man	Manitoba, Canada	Prolymphocytic leukemia	PCR	None	Lane et al., 2000
7	5	F	Identified but not stated	Providence, Rhode Island	Neuroblastoma	Blood smear	Nifurtimox	Saulnier-Sholler et al., 2006

Table 5.3. Transfusion-Transmitted Chagas Disease Cases in the United States and Canada

T. cruzi (4.9%). All were asymptomatic, but the presence of parasites was demonstrated by xenodiagnosis in three out of six examined. The authors estimated that there were at the time between 500,000 and 2 million Central Americans living in the United States and that 5% or as many as 25,000–100,000 may have had chronic Chagas disease.

Kirchhoff (1989) further suggested that additional transfusion-related cases could be occurring in immunocompetent patients that remain undetected due to a more benign course of illness, thus suggesting the possibility that potential donors who have lived in Chagas-endemic countries should be deferred as blood donors. Skolnick (1989, 1991) reviewed the available data and suggested similar considerations, particularly in relation to the deferral policy at blood banks, calling attention to Chagas disease as a new threat to the U.S. blood supply.

Kerndt et al. (1991) performed a serological survey in Los Angeles of 998 donors, 38.5% of them born in endemic areas of Latin America, and 11 of them (1.1%) were seroreactive to *T. cruzi* antigen by CF and/or IIF testing. In a more thorough review of the subject, Kirchhoff (1992) recommended that "prescreening with a questionnaire may be an effective and a relatively simple alternative to serological screening." Appleman et al. (1993) evaluated the usefulness of the questionnaire and observed that 72 of 3,492 donors in California were judged to be at high risk of being infected with *T. cruzi*. Forty-five of these donors were subsequently tested, and two were found to be seropositive. Following a series of discussions about the existence of undiagnosed Chagas disease cases in the United States, mainly among immigrants, Milei et al. (1992) made some quantitative estimations based on the figures presented in the study by Kirchhoff et al. (1987) for Central Americans. On the basis of the total population of immigrants from Latin America residing in the United States, they calculated that about 500,000–675,000 people could be infected and that, of those, approximately 75,000 could suffer chronic cardiomyopathy. They stated that "most of these individuals probably are either undiagnosed or misdiagnosed as having either idiopathic (dilated) cardiomyopathy or coronary artery disease, since Chagas disease is largely unrecognized and blood screening is rarely performed."

Subsequent studies sought to evaluate a new generation of highly sensitive and specific antibody tests, including analysis of risk factor questions as screening tools.

Brashear et al. (1995) tested 13,309 sera from eight blood banks from the western and southwestern United States (New Mexico, Texas, and California) using the Abbott enzyme immunoassay (EIA) test. Of this group of donors, 7,835 were of Latin American origin. Seroreactivity to *T. cruzi* was observed in 14 individuals (0.105%), five of them were from Brazil. To evaluate the effectiveness of risk factor questions, Galel and Kirchhoff (1996) gave a questionnaire to 17,521 donors in 18 participating centers in California, with 57 individuals reporting at least one risk factor related to Chagas disease. However, the authors pointed out that donors could be reluctant to answer the questions honestly. They also considered that "An estimated infection prevalence of 1 in 8,500 is on the same order of magnitude as that of other transfusion-transmissible infections for which serologic screening of blood donors is currently mandated." Finally, they added that "donor screening for *T. cruzi* should be considered seriously." A similar opinion was expressed by Leiby et al. (1997), who had the opportunity to test 49,465 American Red Cross donors from Los Angeles and Orange Counties, California, and from metropolitan Miami (South Florida). Of these donors, 105 (0.21%) were repeat reactive by EIA and 34 were confirmed by RIPA; 33 (0.14%) of those confirmed positive were from the 23,978 people who responded "yes" to the risk factor question, whereas one (0.004%) who confirmed positive was from 25,478 people who responded "no." In the latter situation, it was determined that the only positive case was a person who was born in and had lived in El Salvador. Also, all 34 positive people were either from Latin America or had traveled or worked there. The authors made the following statement: "we estimate that at least 2.5% of blood donors nationwide have geographic risk of exposure to *T. cruzi* with higher rates in certain areas, such as Miami and Los Angeles."

By using a different approach, Barrett et al. (1997) obtained all-negative results by testing sera from 6,013 donors selected at random and collected by the American Red Cross Gulf Coast Region in northwestern Florida, southern Georgia, southern Alabama, and parts of Mississippi and Louisiana. Donor samples were initially screened by indirect hemagglutination, and at least one of the three different EIAs. Eighty-five samples tested positive by one screening method, but only 10 samples tested positive by more than one method. Confirmatory testing of the 85 by RIPA (American Red Cross) revealed that they all were negative.

Shulman et al. (1997), using donors from the Medical Center Blood Bank of Los Angeles County and the University of Southern California, determined that, of 3,320 donors, 1,311 were at risk for *T. cruzi* infection based on an answer to a questionnaire, and, when tested serologically seven were repeat reactive by EIA and six were subsequently confirmed by RIPA. The authors claimed that "The results of the current study demonstrate that eligible blood donors may posses *T. cruzi*-specific antibodies and that a commercially available assay can be used to identify these donors under field conditions in the United States."

Leiby et al. (2002) pointed out that blood donors seropositive for *T. cruzi* (seroprevalence in selected U.S. blood donor population ranges from 0 to 0.48%) could be found throughout the country.

A larger and more comprehensive study conducted by the American Red Cross in Los Angeles and Miami screened over 1.1 million and 181,139 donations, respectively, for risk exposure using a risk question and antibody testing over a 52-month period (Leiby et al., 2002). In Los Angeles, 7.1% of those queried showed a positive response to the risk question, whereas in Miami 14.3% responded affirmatively. Of those tested, a total of 147 in Los Angeles (0.19%) and 20 in Miami (0.08%) were confirmed as seropositive (1 in 7,500 and 1 in 9,000 donations, respectively) (Leiby et al., 2002). In another report, Leiby (2004) stated that "Nationwide estimates indicate that approximately 1 in every 25,000 U.S. blood donors is infected with *T. cruzi* and thus at risk for transmitting the infection to blood recipients." He also added, "Thus, for those non-endemic countries seeking a rational intervention, universal blood screening appears to be the most promising approach to ensure blood safety."

In 2005, a new commercial test manufactured by Ortho-Clinical Diagnostic (Raritan, New Jersey) was developed for screening in blood banks; it was licensed by the Food and Drug Administration in December 2006. It is an ELISA-type test, made with epimastigote lysate antigens, intended for use in blood donation screening and not for clinical diagnosis. The American Red Cross conducted a study with the test in two collection centers in California (Los Angeles and Oakland) and one in Arizona (Tucson), from August 2006 to January 2007. Of a total of 148,969 samples tested, 63 were repeat reactive, and from these 32 (one in 4,655) were confirmed by RIPA. The same test has been used in 10,192 donations from blood donors residing in El Paso, Texas, and in

178 selected blood samples from Latin America. In the first group three reactive samples were found, confirmed by RIPA for a specificity of 100%, and in the second group 173 were reactive, for a sensitivity of 97.7% (Tobler et al., 2007). Since 2007, the test has been recommended for use in all blood banks (Stramer et al., 2007). Initially, most blood centers screened donors universally (i.e., every donation from every donor tested). Within the last year, however, most blood centers have implemented a selective screening strategy whereby donors are only tested once and, if negative, are not retested upon subsequent donations. Donors confirmed as positive are deferred from future donation.

In addition to vectorial and transfusion transmission, *T. cruzi* is also transmissible congenitally and by organ transplantation. To date, systematic studies of congenital transmission in the United States are lacking, and thus estimates of its frequency are unavailable.

However, Leiby et al. (1999) reported the first two possible autochthonous congenital cases in two serologically positive blood donors born in the United States; neither reportedly had traveled to any endemic area nor had other risk factors for infection. In both the cases, family history revealed that they had Mexican ancestors with antecedents of heart ailments compatible with Chagas disease.

In a serological survey of 2,107 Hispanic and 1,658 non-Hispanic pregnant women attending Houston City Health Clinics (1993–1996), Di Pentima et al. (1999) found *T. cruzi* antibody prevalences of 0.4% and 0.1% (respectively) using two serological tests (ELISA and IHA). On the basis of seroprevalence obtained in the survey and the conservative estimate of congenital transmission occurring in 1–4% of pregnancies, Di Pentima et al. (1999) estimated that about 10–40 cases of transplacental transmission of Chagas disease could occur annually in Texas.

Buekens et al. (2008) estimated the number of newborns congenitally infected with *T. cruzi* in North America, based on the scarce seroprevalence data available from Canada, Mexico, and the United States. In spite of the imprecise numbers, as recognized by the authors, they concluded that 2,028 newborns are likely to be congenitally infected in North America and that, of these, 189 infections will occur annually in the United States.

Yadon and Schmuñis (2009) called attention to the potential risk of congenital Chagas disease among immigrant women of childbearing age from endemic countries who are living in the United States. Considering the prevalence rates in their respective countries and the degree of risk of a newborn of becoming infected, based on two different census years (1990 and 2000), the authors were able to estimate the potential number of infected children who acquired congenital Chagas disease (85–318 in 1990 and 166–635 in 2000). In spite of the authors' recognition of the limitations of the parameters on which they based their assumption, they stated that "congenital transmission might be more important than is recognized in the United States." Therefore, they recommended that health professionals should pay special attention to this potential problem.

Verani et al. (2010) surveyed practicing obstetricians and gynecologists to measure their knowledge of Chagas disease and the risk of congenital transmission. Among those who responded to the questionnaire, the majority confessed to having "very limited" knowledge or having "never heard of it." On the basis of their data, the authors suggest that "a greater awareness of Chagas disease may help to detect treatable congenital cases in the United States."

In contrast to congenital transmission, transmission or reactivation of the chronic phase of Chagas disease by organ transplantation in the United States is better understood; this has particularly been so during the past two decades. Libow et al. (1991) made reference to the potential of reactivation of Chagas disease following cardiac transplantation in patients with Chagasic cardiomyopathy. They mentioned the previous experience in São Paulo, Brazil, where three of four patients receiving heart transplants experienced reactivation of the disease. In the Brazilian cases, the "new" acute phase had certain peculiarities; for example, the parasitological and serological tests failed to reveal *T. cruzi* infection, while the patients showed a skin rash on the lower limbs and/or thorax from which parasites could be obtained (Stolf et al., 1987). A fifth patient, a 22-year-old man from Honduras who had a heart transplant at the Columbia University Presbyterian Medical Center, New York, developed congestive heart failure with cardiomegaly at onset; the ECG revealed a first-degree heart block, left anterior hemiblock, and RBBB, and his ejection fraction was 14%. He also had a positive ELISA test for *T. cruzi* antibodies. Five months after the cardiac transplant, he revealed marked dilation of all chambers with aneurismal dilation of both apices. A skin biopsy of an erythematous plaque (cellulites) in the right thigh revealed amastigotes of *T. cruzi*. After a diagnosis of reactivated

Chagas disease, the patient was treated with nifurtimox, prednisone, and cyclosporine, and, in spite of some complications, he was discharged after improvement and 18 months later his condition was satisfactory (Libow et al., 1991).

Tanowitz et al. (1992) discussed the situation presented by several cases of reactivation of Chagas disease in HIV-infected patients (see next section) and additional cases caused by organ transplantation. They claimed that "since the number of hearts available for transplantation is only a small percentage of the number of potential recipients, *T. cruzi* infection should be considered a contraindication for heart transplantation because of the likelihood of serious posttransplant complications related to reactivation of the parasitosis." Similarly, Kirchhoff (1993) made reference to the six known cases of Chagas patients who had had cardiac transplantation in the United States up to that date. Three of them experienced reactivation of infection, but in the other three this was avoided by using a prophylactic treatment with nifurtimox.

By using a different approach, Leiby et al. (2000) focused on the problem by looking at the presence of *T. cruzi* in patients undergoing cardiac surgery, including a subpopulation of immigrants. The study was designed to assess transfusion transmission, but no evidence of transfusion-transmitted *T. cruzi* was found. Six postoperative patients out of 11,430 samples available were confirmed to be serologically positive by two tests (EIA and RIPA) and, of these, five were Hispanic. Two of the six seropositive patients had received heart transplants; the parasite was confirmed by a PCR test in preserved heart tissues. Out of 184 Hispanics enrolled in the study, 2.7% were seropositive for *T. cruzi*.

To date, five cases of *T. cruzi* transmission by organ transplantation have been reported in the United States. Zayas et al. (2002) reported on what they considered to be the first three proven cases of organ transplantation transmission in the United States. All three recipients received cadaveric organs from the same donor, an immigrant from Central America. The first woman, aged 37 years, received one kidney and the pancreas; the second, aged 32, received the liver; and the third, aged 69, received the other kidney. In all the three patients, parasites were confirmed in their blood by culture. Despite treatment with nifurtimox, the first patient, who was the most immunosuppressed, died of acute chagasic myocarditis; the liver recipient died from other causes, but the third case responded satisfactorily to treatment.

Mascola et al. (2006) and Kun et al. (2009) reported two additional cases of transmission by solid organ transplantation. The first was in a 64-year-old man who had received a heart transplant. Subsequently, *T. cruzi* was identified in his blood and the parasitemia was controlled with nifurtimox; nevertheless, the man died as a result of acute cellular rejection. The donor was a Hispanic male who was born in the United States and traveled to an endemic area of Mexico. This donor yielded a seropositive test for *T. cruzi* antibodies. The donor's mother was born in Mexico but attempts to interview or test her were unsuccessful. The second case involved a 73-year-old male patient who also had received a heart transplant. Following complaints of fever and fatigue, he was readmitted. *T. cruzi* was demonstrated in a peripheral blood smear. In spite of treatment with nifurtimox, he died of cardiac failure 25 weeks after surgery. The organ donor was a Salvadoran immigrant who was serologically positive at death.

These cases have raised concerns about the safety of donated organs. Nowicki et al. (2006) serologically tested 404 serum samples from deceased organ donors in the Southern California area. They found three Hispanic donors whose test results were positive for *T. cruzi* antibodies, using an EIA commercial test, and one of them was confirmed by IFAT at the CDC. The authors raised the question of the need for screening organ donors from endemic countries as a means to prevent transmission of Chagas disease through organ transplantation.

5.4 CHAGAS DISEASE IN IMMIGRANTS

It is a well-known fact that Chagas disease is now present in non-endemic areas of the world such as Europe, Japan, and Australia. Infected Latin American immigrants have created a new threat through the human-to-human mechanisms of transmission, mainly blood transfusion (Coura and Albajar-Viñas, 2010; Gascon et al., 2010; Tanowitz et al., 2011).

In this section, we will summarize some specific information available about cases of Chagas disease with different pathologies that have been encountered among Latin American immigrants in the United States. This constitutes further evidence that chronic Chagas disease occurs in several areas of the United States among people who have migrated from areas where the disease is endemic.

Scherb and Arias (1962) reported a case of achalasia of the esophagus that was attributed to Chagas disease in a 52-year-old woman who was born in Guayaquil, Ecuador, and who had been living in the United States for the previous 8 years. The woman was admitted to the Bronx Municipal Center because of intermittent dysphagia and loss of weight, and she showed a positive serological test (CF) for *T. cruzi*.

Massumi and Gooch (1965) studied a similar case in a native 46-year-old Brazilian woman, with achalasia and megaesophagus, associated with myocarditis, who was admitted to the George Washington Medical Division of the District of Columbia General Hospital. She had diffuse cardiomegaly and an altered ECG with abnormal P waves, first-degree A-V block, ventricular premature beats, and a complete right branch block (CRBBB) with left axis deviation. The CF test was positive for *T. cruzi*.

Lorenzana (1967) related the case of a 55-year-old man who was born and spent the first 2 months of his life in Argentina, then being taken to Italy and later migrating to the United States at the age of 21. He was admitted to the Washington Hospital Center, Washington D.C., with facial paralysis and left hemiplegia, and died as a consequence of hemorrhagic infarction of the brain. At the autopsy, a chronic myocarditis was found, with amastigote forms in the heart muscle and a mural thrombus in the apex of the left ventricle. This is an interesting case because, as the authors stated, it is difficult to know whether the patient had had a dormant *T. cruzi* infection for many years or whether the infection had been acquired in the United States.

A similar case, with cardiomyopathy and cerebral embolism causing hemiplegia, was observed in a 49-year-old Ecuadorian female who had resided in Brooklyn, New York, for 8 years. The patient came to the Lutheran Medical Center in 1975 and showed a bizarre ECG, and the CF and IHA tests were positive for Chagas disease (Shafi, 1977).

A 23-year-old woman from El Salvador, after living in the United States for 3 years, was referred to the Los Angeles County-University of Southern California Medical Center with arrhythmias. Other heart abnormalities included ventricular extrasystoles and ventricular tachycardia with apical left ventricular cardiac aneurysm. The IHA reaction for *T. cruzi* was positive (Edmiston et al., 1978).

A chronic Chagas disease case was diagnosed in California in a 75-year-old woman who had lived 30 years earlier in El Salvador. She had a progressive congestive cardiomyopathy in the absence of hypertension, an

RBBB, and sinus bradycardia. Several CF tests were performed, yielding positive results for *T. cruzi*. At the autopsy, there was diffuse myocarditis but parasites were not found (Pearlman, 1983).

An 86-year-old Ecuadorian man, who emigrated to the United States when he was 25, was admitted to the Brooklyn Veteran Administration Medical Center in New York because of chest pain and was diagnosed with coronary artery disease. The patient had no evidence of heart failure and had a normal-size heart and ECG evidence of a prior lateral infarction (Q wave). A serological test for Chagas disease (CF) was positive. The authors of this case report (Feit et al., 1983) stated the following: "The North American inexperience with Chagas disease may often cause it to be overlooked. A recent review of pseudoinfarction Q waves failed even to mention Chagas disease. We strongly recommend that Chagas disease always be included in the differential diagnosis."

Kirchhoff and Neva (1985) discussed three Bolivian cases of Chagas disease studied at the National Institutes of Health in Bethesda. The patients, all males, aged 37, 38, and 35, had positive serological tests for *T. cruzi* infection. The first patient was asymptomatic upon presentation, the second showed megacolon and a CRBBB, and the last had a complete heart block and cerebral vascular involvement with left hemiparesis and expressive aphasia of embolic origin. The authors alerted physicians to these cardinal features of chronic Chagas disease.

From 1974 to 1990, Hagar and Rahimtoola (1991) analyzed the case histories of patients at the Los Angeles County-University of Southern California Medical Center who had a positive serological test for *T. cruzi*. The authors selected 25 patients from several Latin American countries (seven men and 18 women) with no evidence of obstructive coronary artery disease and who they considered to have Chagas heart disease. They presented the cardiologic characteristics of these patients and the initial ECG findings and stated that "congestive heart failure ($p = 0.0002$) and the presence of either left ventricular aneurysm or left ventricular dysfunction ($p = 0.003$) were the only independent predictions of subsequent death." The authors concluded that "Our study provides useful clinical information on the presentation, clinical features and outcome of the disease."

Gluckstein et al. (1992) reported the case of a 32-year-old HIV-infected Salvadoran homosexual man, living in Los Angeles, who was admitted to the hospital with fever, right-sided weakness, aphasia, and decreased visual acuity. A mass was discovered at the left temporal lobe, and a biopsy showed intracellular amastigotes that were successfully cultured. This is the first brain abscess due to infection with *T. cruzi* reported in the United States, and only a few others have been reported from South America. A similar case from Argentina in a 19-year-old man with hemophilia and AIDS who had a reactivation of Chagas disease with a tumor-like lesion of the brain was reported by Del Castillo et al. (1990). Another interesting case was that of a 48-year-old woman from Campinas, São Paulo, Brazil, with AIDS and right-side hemiplegia. Typanosomes were observed in the CSF and amastigotes were detected in the brain at autopsy (Metze and Maciel, 1993).

Ciesielski et al. (1993), in a serological survey of 99 immigrant farm workers from Latin America living in North Carolina, found that two Mexican-born people were seropositive for *T. cruzi*, but unfortunately the authors did not follow up on these individuals. We should also mention a fatal case in a 13-month-old girl who immigrated to Canada from Paraguay and died of acute myocarditis caused by *T. cruzi* infection. At the autopsy, parasites were observed in the myocardial fibers and in the smooth muscle of the esophagus and larynx (Montalvo-Hicks et al., 1980).

Holbert et al. (1995) reported a case of a 61-year-old Brazilian woman, seen at the Singing River Hospital System at Ocean Springs, Mississippi, with cardiomyopathy and congestive heart failure, and a serological positive titer for Chagas disease.

In a recent paper, Bern and Montgomery (2009) used published seroprevalence data from 18 Latin American countries to estimate the number of immigrants with Chagas disease infection among the 22.8 million living in the United States. They produced a figure of 300,167 people infected with *T. cruzi* and calculated that between 30,000 and 45,000 had cardiomyopathy and that around 63–315 newborns had acquired congenital infection. Even though the authors recognize the various "sources of uncertainty" in these figures, they call attention to the need to improve assessment of the real impact of Chagas disease among immigrants.

After a careful appraisal of the burden represented by infected immigrants from Latin American endemic areas, a group of 14 specialists from South and North America have provided some practical recommendations for "evaluation, counseling and etiological treatment of patients." Treatment with the available drugs (nifurtimox and benznidazole) should be offered to persons 18 years or younger and to patients with acute disease, including early congenital infections and reactivations in patients with AIDS or other types of immunosuppression. This treatment should also be offered to patients aged 19–50 years without advanced heart disease, and for those older than 50 years without advanced cardiomyopathy the treatment should be optional (Bern et al., 2007). In a second paper (Bern et al. 2008), the authors reaffirm previous concepts stressing the importance of widespread bloodbank screening to prevent transfusion transmission, and they continue to recommend the same etiological treatment criteria presented previously.

5.5 LABORATORY-ACQUIRED INFECTIONS

A few accidental laboratory infections with *T. cruzi* have occurred in the United States, and at least four of these cases have appeared in the literature. Aronson (1962) related the case of a 22-year-old microbiologist who spilled a suspension of the Chilean Tulahuen strain of *T. cruzi* on his left hand and became infected apparently through a skin abrasion in one of his fingers. The patient was admitted to the Chenango Memorial Hospital in New York, where a mixed infection of *Neisseria perflava* and *T. cruzi* was demonstrated by blood culture.

Another accidental case in a 58-year-old laboratory technician who had worked with the Tulahuen strain for more than 20 years, was reported by Western et al. (1969), from the CDC in Atlanta, Georgia. The patient showed a chagoma of the left thumb and other symptoms such as fever, malaise, and transient pedal edema. The blood cultures were positive for *T. cruzi*, as were two serological reactions (CF and IHA). She improved upon treatment with Bayer 2502, and, subsequently, her cultures became negative and her antibody titers declined.

Hanson et al. (1974) were able to study the immunoglobulin concentrations and antibody response, at different times after the accident, in an acute laboratory-acquired case of Chagas disease. This case occurred in an American scientist who punctured his finger with a needle when it was being used to infect mice with a Brazilian strain of *T. cruzi*. Clinical signs appeared after 16–18 days, and this patient was also treated with Bayer 2502. There was an evident remission, and the levels of IgM and IgG came close to the original levels at day 159 after the inoculation.

Another case occurred in a 28-year-old medical technician admitted to the Bronson Methodist Hospital in Kalamazoo, Michigan, with fever and myalgia. He also showed lymphadenopathy, splenomegaly, and an

ECG consistent with acute myocarditis. Parasites were revealed in fresh blood, and this patient responded well to nifurtimox. The infection occurred when he was dissecting a mouse infected with the Tulahuen strain *T. cruzi* without wearing gloves; he apparently had a break in the skin at a nail margin, which provided a site of entry for the parasite (Cerovski, 1980).

Brener (1984) reviewed the cases of laboratory-acquired Chagas disease reported in the literature as well as cases known through personal contacts. He was able to identify, up to that date, about 45 cases in Latin America, Europe, and the United States. He recommended that treatment with a drug such as nifurtimox begin immediately following an accident.

More recently, Herwaldt (2001) also reviewed these laboratory accidents for several diseases. With respect to laboratory-acquired *T. cruzi* infections, she compiled 65 cases from around the world and presented some details about the years of occurrence, geographical distribution, routes of exposure, and clinical manifestations. The statistical figures presented indicated that eight of the 65 cases had occurred in the United States.

CHAPTER 6

Final Remarks

Compiling the scattered and at times incomplete literature published in journals of different disciplines, or in other types of publications, has been a useful exercise in understanding what is really known about Chagas disease in the United States. There is historical evidence showing that the insect vectors have existed in the United States for several centuries and have been observed both in wild conditions and in visiting human dwellings. It is also known that the parasite that produces the disease, *T. cruzi*, has been in the country for a very long time, as demonstrated by the great genetic diversity found. *T. cruzi* was first found in a Californian bug (*T. protracta*) only a few years following Carlos Chagas' discovery in Brazil, though it was not accurately identified at that time.

Today in the United States, 11 species of Chagas disease vectors are present not only in the southern parts of the country, as previously believed, but also in the middle and northeast regions, in a total of 27 states. Some species such as *T. lecticularia* and *T. sanguisuga* are widely distributed (16 and 23 states, respectively), whereas others are restricted to certain areas and tend to be scarce. At least seven species have been found in or near houses in 12 states, and six of them are reported to have colonized human dwellings, completing the life cycle in houses, although generally in small numbers. This situation leads us to think that more careful searches, particularly in areas where there are houses with poor sanitary conditions, will probably yield colonies with more than a few bugs of some of these species. Yet, the common visits by adult bugs to many households in certain areas of the country, particularly during the warm months of the year, need more attention due to their potential epidemiological implications.

The finding of eight species of bugs infected with *T. cruzi* in at least 10 states, with mean infection prevalence of *T. cruzi* similar to those found in Latin America, indicates that, under certain circumstances, vectorial transmission is possible and could take place at a higher rate than previously believed. Special attention should be given to areas of Arizona, where *T. rubida* and *T. recurva* are frequent visitors to homes. In certain

An Appraisal of the Status of Chagas Disease in the United States. DOI: 10.1016/B978-0-12-397268-2.00006-7

parts of Texas, *T. gerstaeckeri* and *T. lecticularia* are commonly found close to humans. In areas of California and New Mexico, *T. protracta* is a good invader of homes, and in Alabama, Georgia, and Louisiana *T. sanguisuga* has frequently been found in domestic habitats.

The classical factors that previously led Chagas disease being considered as a Latin American illness can no longer be substantiated. The expansion of settlements and other incursions into formerly wild areas, plus the social deterioration of housing conditions in certain localities in the United States, facilitate contact with wild kissing bugs, thus stimulating their capacity to thrive in houses. Conversely, the assertion that the American species are slow defecators might not always be true, particularly, in some areas of the country where they seem to act as rather efficient vectors. This leads us to believe that vectorial transmission is regularly taking place in some areas, making them endemic pockets, in spite of rather low morbidity indexes.

The association of eight species of triatomines with wood rats of the genus *Neotoma* in at least eight states is a common biological fact. This is probably a very old relationship that has been maintained for centuries, attaining a good level of equilibrium particularly for the insects and for the parasite transmitted by them, with important epidemiological significance. The rats serve as permanent hosts and as reservoirs for the trypanosome, becoming easily infected when they eat the bugs but without being markedly affected. Infected bugs, particularly adults, are seasonally attracted to lights in human-made ecotopes and may move from this well-established wild cycle to start a domestic cycle of the disease involving other mammals such as dogs and, in a few cases, humans. It is estimated that the majority of these bugs complete their life cycle (egg to adult) in the dens of the wood rats in about 1 year, as observed in the laboratory for some species. More detailed studies on the cycles and behavior of the main species are needed, under controlled laboratory conditions as well as under natural conditions.

As a consequence of adult bugs entering homes, a phenomenon that has been well-known for far more than a century, serious local and systemic reactions have been observed on various occasions in people bitten by the bugs. Anaphylactic reactions, which in some cases can lead to very serious and even life-threatening situations, do not occur, or are considered exceptional, in Latin America. This is probably due to the different relationship existing between humans and bugs in this region, compared to the United States. In the latter, there is mainly seasonal contact with humans, in an intermittent fashion, whereas in Latin America the contact is more permanent and constant. In the first case, individuals become sensitized to the bugs' salivary substances and, when bitten again, after a longer interval, an anaphylactic reaction is more likely to be triggered. In the second situation, there are opportunities for desensitization when people receive repeated bites at shorter intervals. This hypothesis is feasible, based on empirical facts, and supported at least partially by clinical and epidemiological observations as well as by experimental desensitization tests with bugs' salivary gland extracts. Nevertheless, more extensive work on possible differences in the composition of the saliva of bugs from different geographical areas is necessary to clarify whether one or more particular substances are responsible for the anaphylactic reactions.

With respect to animal reservoirs by demonstration of the parasites' presence, several reports show that at least 18 different species of mammals are found naturally infected with the parasite in the United States, distributed across 14 states, and three other species have been detected by serological methods. Two of these, opossums and raccoons, are more widely distributed and are commonly infected by *T. cruzi* in seven and nine states, respectively. These two wild reservoirs are frequently found close to humans and could play an important epidemiological role, as in the case of wood rats, by linking the wild cycle of the parasite with a domestic one. Opossums, in particular, seem to play this role due to the frequency with which they become associated with humans in certain areas of the house such as attics, cellars, or even in the crawl spaces beneath floors. Moreover, opossums can also carry the insect infectious form of the parasite.

The role of dogs as domestic reservoirs deserves special mention. They present clinical symptoms similar to those of humans, with the characteristic acute and chronic phases of the disease. They frequently ingest bugs and are easily infected by this oral route. The fact that dogs with parasitologicaly confirmed infections have been detected in at least five states, and in 11 more by serology, suggesting that the problem is underestimated. It is important to realize that dogs can serve as a source of infection for other bugs if they are present in a domestic environment. Some of the pathological changes observed in dogs naturally or experimentally infected with North American strains of *T. cruzi* are very similar to those produced by Latin American strains, including ECG changes, which mimic those observed in humans, showing that some strains are quite pathogenic for these animals. This fact has also been demonstrated in other experimentally infected laboratory animals, proving that low and high virulent strains are present in the United States.

The prevalence of Chagas disease in the United States is low in comparison to what is seen in Latin America, but, due to its clinical characteristics and due to the lack of knowledge by physicians in some areas, it is probably underestimated. In fact, during the first half of the 20th century, Chagas disease was assumed to be absent from the United States and considered an exotic disease until the first two indigenous cases were discovered, almost simultaneously, in Texas in 1955. To these, four more cases, attributed to local vectorial transmission, have been added (one more in Texas, one in California, one in Tennessee, and one in Louisiana), all by fortuitous circumstances. This again indicates that physicians are not aware of the characteristics of the disease and are probably overlooking other locally acquired cases, particularly those with milder clinical symptoms.

In relation to serological prevalence in the country, a few surveys, mainly in areas of Texas and Georgia, also indicate that the rates are low. Nevertheless, new serological surveys are needed among representative human populations, particularly in certain areas of certain states, together with bug searches in and around houses. The trials should be done with more sensitive and specific tests that seek to pinpoint possible endemic areas where vectorial transmission is feasible and may be occurring at low rates.

Transfusion-acquired cases deserve special mention. The confirmation of this type of transmission in five patients, at least four of them immunocompromised, from California, New York, Texas, Florida, and Rhode Island, leads us to believe that other such cases may be overlooked, particularly in immunocompetent people in whom the disease follows a more benign course. This issue has received more attention within the last few years, particularly in the areas where potential donor pools consist of populations from countries where Chagas disease is endemic. The serological surveys already performed in some areas of the country indicate that eligible blood donors from these groups may have *T. cruzi*-specific antibodies and that the estimated prevalence rate is equivalent to that of other transfusion-transmissible agents for which serological screening of blood donors is currently performed. The recent development of a new ELISA screening test, licensed by the FDA, represents a new hope for the use of this test in all blood banks to further enhance the safety of the blood supply in the United States.

With the large number of Latin American immigrants now living in the United States, a new risk has appeared through congenital transmission in childbearing women, a problem that deserves attention.

In some instances, transmission or reactivation of the chronic stage of the disease has been associated with organ transplantation. The first five cases confirmed in the last few years indicate that preventive measures should be taken. Consequently, it is important that the risk of Chagas disease transmission and Chagas-related complications be considered by surgeons performing these services.

In general, physicians in the United States should be aware of the symptoms and characteristics of chronic Chagas disease, particularly in immigrants from Latin America, including the risk of congenital transmission. It seems evident that patients with various symptoms that could be attributed to chronic Chagas disease should seek medical attention in hospitals or clinics. Chagasic myocardiopathy could be misdiagnosed as a coronary or idiopathic artery disease. Chagas disease should also be considered in gastrointestinal tract abnormalities, such as achalasia, megaesophagus, and megacolon (fecaloma, sigmoid volvulus). Additionally, physicians should be aware of the various clinical symptoms that are present in people who have Chagas disease and become infected with HIV or are otherwise immunosuppressed. Furthermore, it is necessary to pay more attention to the risk of acquiring Chagas disease accidentally in the laboratory and, in this respect, to maintain meticulous safety practices in laboratories where the etiologic agent is maintained for research purposes.

Finally, mortality data related to Chagas disease are scarce and/or underestimated in the United States. Herein, we pointed out some examples of death as a consequence of acute and chronic *T. cruzi* infections in both native and migrant individuals. According to the number of infected people living in the country and the proportion expected to have Chagas heart disease, the mortality rate due to this trypanosomiasis must be higher than estimated, but is not being registered due to a failure in medical diagnosis and lack of expertise.

ACKNOWLEDGMENTS

The senior author received partial support from the ChagaSpace Project. We thank Dr. Ellen Dotson (Centers for Disease Control and Prevention, Atlanta, GA) for providing some of the older papers to the senior author. The photographs were obtained by courtesy of the photographers Margarethe Brummermann, Harold Baquet, Mike Quinn, and Michael Schumacher.

REFERENCES

Adams, R.R., Ryckman, R.E., 1969. A comparative electrophoresis study of the *Triatoma rubida* complex (Hemiptera: Reduviidae: Triatominae). J. Med. Entomol. 6, 1–18.

Africa, C.M., 1934. Three cases of poisonous insect bite involving *Triatoma rubrofasciata*. Phillipp. J. Sci. 53, 169–176.

Anonymous, 1938. Chagas' Disease. Annual report of the Surgeon General of U.S. Public Health Service Goverment Printing Office, Washington, D.C. pp. 56–57.

Anonymous, 1955. National Office of Vital Statistics: Communicable Diseases Summary for Week Ended December 10, 1955. U.S. Department of Health, Education, and Welfare, Washington, D.C. pp. 2–3.

Anonymous, 1956. Found: Two cases of chagas' disease. Texas Health Bull. 9, 11–13.

Appleman, M.D., Shulman, I.A., Saxena, S.D., Kirchhoff, L.V., 1993. Use of a questionnaire to identify potential blood donors at risk for infection with *Trypanosoma cruzi*. Transfus. 33, 61–64.

Arnold, H.L., Bell, D.B., 1944. Kissing bug bites. J. Allergy Clin. Immunol. 74, 436–442.

Aronson, P.R., 1962. Septicemia from concomitant infection with *Trypanosoma cruzi* and *Neisseria perflava*: First case of laboratory-acquired Chagas' disease in the U.S. Ann. Intl. Med. 57, 994–1000.

Balazuc, J., 1950. Un fenómeno de anafilaxia producido por picaduras de Triatoma (Hemiptera: Reduviidae). An. Inst. Med. Reg. (Universidad Nacional de Tacumán) 3, 35–37.

Barnabé, C., Yeager, R., Pung, O., Tibayrenc, M., 2001. *Trypanosoma cruzi*: A considerable phylogenetic divergence indicates that the agent of Chagas disease is indigenous to the native fauna of the United States. Exp. Parasitol. 99, 73–79.

Barr, S.C., Baker, D., Markovits, J., 1986. Trypanosomiasis and laryngeal paralysis in a dog. J. Am. Vet. Med. Assoc. 88, 1307–1309.

Barr, S.C., Simpson, R.M., Schmidt, S.P., Bunge, M.M., Authement, J.M., Lozano, F., 1989. Chronic dilatative myocarditis caused by *Trypanosoma cruzi* in two dogs. J. Am. Vet. Med. Assoc. 195, 1237–1241.

Barr, S.C., Brown, C., Dennis, V.A., Klei, T.R., 1990a. Infections of inbred mice with three *Trypanosoma cruzi* isolates from Louisiana mammals. J. Parasitol. 76, 918–921.

Barr, S.C., Dennis, V.A., Klei, T.R., 1990b. Growth characteristics in axenic and cell cultures, protein profiles and zymodeme typing of three *Trypanosoma cruzi* isolates from Louisiana mammals. J. Parasitol. 76, 631–638.

Barr, S.C., Brown, C.C., Dennis, V.A., Klei, T.R., 1991a. The lesions and prevalence of *Trypanosoma cruzi* in opossums and armadillos from Southern Louisiana. J. Parasitol. 77, 624–627.

Barr, S.C., Gossett, K.A., Klei, T.R., 1991b. Clinical, clinico-pathologic and parasitologic observations of trypanosomiasis in dogs infected with North American *Trypanosoma cruzi* isolates. Am. J. Vet. Res. 52, 954–960.

Barr, S.C., Schmidt, S.P., Brown, C.C., Klei, T.R., 1991c. Pathologic features of dogs inoculated with North American *Trypanosoma cruzi* isolates. Am. J. Vet. Res. 52, 2033–2039.

Barr, S.C., Dennis, V.A., Klei, T.R., 1991d. Serologic and blood culture survey of *Trypanosoma cruzi* infection in four canine populations of southern Louisiana. Am. J. Vet. Res. 52, 570–573.

Barr, S.C., Dennis, V.A., Klei, T.R., Norcross, N.L., 1991e. Antibody and lymphoblastogenic responses of dogs experimentally infected with *Trypanosoma cruzi* isolates from North American mammals. Vet. Immunol. Immunopathol. 29, 267–283.

Barr, S.C., Holmes, R.A., Klei, T.R., 1992. Electrocardiographic and echocardiographic features of trypanosomiasis in dogs inoculated with North American *Trypanosoma cruzi* isolates. Am. J. Vet. Res. 53, 521–527.

Barr, S.C., Van Beek, O., Carlisle-Nowak, M.J., López, J.W., Kirchhoff, L.V., Allison, N., Zajac, A., de Lahunta, A., Schlafer, D.H., Crandall, W.T., 1995. *Trypanosoma cruzi* infection in Walker hounds from Virginia. Am. J. Vet. Res. 56, 1037–1044.

Barrett, V.J., Leiby, D.A., Odom, J.L., Otani, M.M., Rowe, J.D., Roote, J.T., Cox, K.F., Barretto, M.P., 1979. Epidemiologia. In: Brener, Z., Andrade, Z.A. (Eds.), Trypanosoma cruzi e *Doença de Chagas*. Rio de Janeiro, Guanabara Koogan, pp. 89–151.

Beard, C.B., Young, D.G., Butler, J.F., Evans, D.A., 1988. First isolation of *Trypanosoma cruzi* from a wild-caught *Triatoma sanguisuga* (Le Conte) (Hemiptera: Triatominae) in Florida. U.S.A. J. Parasitol. 74, 343–344.

Beard, C.B., Pye, G., Steurer, F.J., Rodríguez, R., Campman, R., Peterson, A.T., Ramsey, J., Wirtz, R.A., Robinson, L.E., 2003. Chagas disease in a domestic transmission cycle in Southern Texas, U.S.A. Emerg. Inf. Dis. 9, 103–105.

Berger, S.L., Palmer, R.H., Hodges, C.C., Hall, G., 1991. Neurologic manifestations of trypanosomiasis in a dog. J. Am. Vet. Med. Assoc. 198, 132–134.

Bern, C., Montgomery, S.P., Herwaldt, B.L., Rassi Jr., A., Marin-Neto, J.A., Dantas, R.O., Maguire, J.H., Acquatella, H., Morillo, C., Kirchhoff, L.V., Gilman, R.H., Reyes, P.A., Salvatella, R., Moore, A.C., 2007. Evaluation and treatment of Chagas disease in the United States. A systematic review. JAMA. 298, 2171–2181.

Bern, C., Montgomery, S.P., Katz, L., Caglioti, S., Stramer, S.L., 2008. Chagas disease and the US blood supply. Curr. Opin. Inf. Dis. 21, 476–482.

Bern, C., Montgomery, S.P., 2009. An estimate of the burden of Chagas disease in the United States. Clin. Inf. Dis. 49, 52–54.

Bice, D.E., 1966. The incidence of *Trypanosoma cruzi* in Triatoma of Tucson. Arizona. Rev. Biol. Trop. 14, 3–12.

Bommineni, Y.R., Dick Jr., E.J., Estep, J.S., Van de Berg, J.L., Hubbard, G.B., 2009. Fatal acute Chagas disease in a chimpanzee. J. Med. Primatol. 38, 247–251.

Bradley, K.K., Bergman, D.K., Woods, J.P., Crutcher, J.M., Kirchhoff, L.V., 2000. Prevalence of American trypanosomiasis (Chagas disease) among dogs in Oklahoma. J. Am. Vet. Med. Assoc. 217, 1853–1857.

Brashear, R.J., Winkler, M.A., Schur, J.D., Lee, H., Burczak, J.D., Hall, H.J., Pan, A.A., 1995. Detection of antibodies to *Trypanosoma cruzi* among blood donors in the southwestern and western United States. I. Evaluation of the sensitivity and specificity of an enzyme immunoassay for detecting antibodies to *Trypanosoma cruzi*. Transfus. 35, 213–218.

Brener, Z., 1973. Biology of *Trypanosoma cruzi*. Ann. Rev. Microbiol. 27, 347–382.

Brener, Z., 1984. Laboratory- acquired Chagas' disease: An endemic disease among parasitologies? In: Morel, C.M. (Ed.), *Genes and Antigens of Parasites. A Laboratory Manual*, second ed. Fundação Oswaldo Cruz, Rio de Janeiro, Brazil, pp. 3–9.

Brooke, M.M., Norman, L., Allain, D., Gorman, G.W., 1957. Isolations of *Trypanosoma cruzi* – like organisms from wild animals collected in Georgia. J. Parasitol. 43 (5, Sec. 2), 15.

Brown, E.L., Roelling, D.M., Gompper, M.E., Monello, R.J., Wenning, K.M., Gabriel, M.W., Yabsley, M.J., 2010. Seroprevalence of *Trypanosoma cruzi* among eleven potential reservoir species from six states across the southern United States. Vect. Borne Zoonot. Dis. 10, 757–763.

Brown, K.R., Hoiles, J.A., Saéz-Alquézar, A., Turrens, J.F., 1997. Negligible prevalence and antibodies against *Trypanosoma cruzi* among blood donors in the southeastern United States. Am. J. Clin. Pathol. 108, 499–503.

Brumpt, E., 1914. Importante du cannibalisme et de le coprophagie chez les *Réduvidés hématophages* (Rhodnius, Triatoma) pour le conservation des Trypanosomes pathogènes en dehors de l' hôte vertébré. Bull. Soc. Pathol. Exot. 7, 702–705.

Buekens, P., Almendares, O., Carlier, Y., Dumonteil, E., Eberhard, M., Gamboa-León, R., James, M., Padilla, N., Wesson, D., Xiong, X., 2008. Mother-to-child transmission of Chagas disease in North America: Why don't we do more? Matern. Child Health J. 12, 283–286.

Burkholder, J.E., Allison, T.C., Kelly, V.P., 1980. *Trypanosoma cruzi* (Chagas) (Protozoa: Kinetoplastida) in invertebrate, reservoir and human hosts of the lower Rio Grande Valley of Texas. J. Parasitol. 66, 305–311.

Carcavallo, R.V., Curto de Casas, S.I., Sherlock, I.A., Galíndez-Girón, I., Jurberg, J., Galvao, C., Mena-Segura, C.A., Noireau, F., 1999. Geographical distribution and alti-latitudinal dispersión. In: Carcavallo, R.V., Galíndez-Girón, I., Jurberg, J., Lent, H. (Eds.), *Atlas of Chagas' Disease Vectors in the Americas*, vol. III. Editora Fiocruz, Rio de Janeiro, Brazil, pp. 747–792.

Cerovski, J.T., 1980. Chagas' disease-Michigan. MMWR. Morb. Mortal. Wkly. Rep. 29, 147–148.

Cesa, K., Caillouët, A., Dorn, P.L., Wesson, D.M., 2011. High *Trypanosoma cruzi* (Kinetoplastida: Trypanosomatidae) prevalence in *Triatoma sanguisuga* (Hemiptera: Reduviidae) in southeastern Louisiana. J. Med. Entomol. 48, 1091–1094.

Chagas, C., 1909a. Uber eine neue Tripanosomiasis des Menschen. Arch. f. Schiffs-u Trop. Hyg. 13, 351–353.

Chagas, C., 1909b. Nova tripanosomiase humana. Estudos sôbre a morfología e o ciclo evolutivo do Schizotrypanum cruzi n. gen., n. sp., ajente etiológicо de nova entidade morbida do homen. Mem. Inst. Osw. Cruz. 1, 159–218.

Chagas, C., 1912. Sôbre um trypanosoma do tatu Tatusia novemcinta, transmitido pelo Triatoma geniculata Latr. (1811). Possibilidade de ser o tatu um depositario do *Trypanosoma cruzi* no mundo exterior. Brasil. Med. 26, 305–306.

Chapman, M.D., Marshall, N.A., Saxon, A., 1986. Identification and partial purification of species-specific allergens from *Triatoma protracta* (Heteroptera: Reduviidae). J. Allergy Clin. Immunol. 74, 436–442.

Cicmanec, J.L., Neva, F.A., McClure, H.M., Locb, W.F., 1974. Accidental infection of laboratory-reared *Macaca mulatta* with *Trypanosoma cruzi*. Lab. Anim. Sci. 24, 783–787.

Ciesielski, S., Seed, J.R., Estrada, J., Wrenn, E., 1993. The seroprevalence of cysticercosis, malaria and *Trypanosoma cruzi* among North Carolina migrant farm workers. Public Health Rep. 108, 736–741.

Cimo, P.L., Luper, W.E., Scouros, M.A., 1993. Transfusion-associated Chagas' disease in Texas: Report of a case. Texas Med. 89, 48–50.

Clark, C.G., Pung, O.J., 1994. Host specificity of ribosomal DNA variation in sylvatic *Trypanosoma cruzi* from North America. Mol. Bioch. Parasitol. 66, 175–179.

Costa, C.H.N., Costa, M.T., Weber, J.N., Gilks, G.F., Castro, C., Marsden, P.D., 1981. Skin reactions to bug bites as a result of xenodiagnosis. Trans. Roy. Soc. Trop. Med. Hyg. 35, 405–408.

Coura, J.R., 1997. *Síntese histórica* e evolução dos conhecimentos sôbre a doença de Chagas. In: Pinto Dias, J.C., Coura, J.R. (Eds.), *Clinica e Terapêutica da doença de Chagas*. Editora Fiocruz, Rio de Janeiro, Brazil, pp. 469–486.

Coura, J.R., Albajar-Viñas, P., 2010. Chagas disease: A new worldwide challenge. Nature. 465, S6–S7.

Cruz-Reyes, A., Pickering-López, J.M., 2006. Chagas disease in Mexico: An analysis of geographical distribution during the past 76 years – A review. Mem. Inst. Osw. Cruz. 101, 345–354.

Cura, C.I., Mejía-Jaramillo, A.M., Duffy, T., Burgos, J.M., Rodriguero, M., Cardinal, M.V., Kjos, S., Gurgel-Gonçalves, R., Blanchet, D., De Pablos, L.M., Tomasini, N., da Silva, A., Russomando, G., Cuba, C.A., Aznar, C., Abate, T., Levin, M.J., Osuna, A., Gürtler, R.E., Diosque, P., Solari, A., Triana-Chávez, O., Schijman, A.G., 2010. *Trypansoma cruzi* I genotypes in different geographical regions and transmission cycles based on a microsatellite motif of the intergenic spacer of spliced-leader genes. Intl. J. Parasitol. 40, 1599–1607.

Davis, D.J., 1943. Infection in monkeys with strains of *Trypanosoma cruzi* isolated in the United States. Public Health Rep. 59, 1006–1010.

Davis, D.J., McGregor, T., de Shazo, T., 1943. *Triatoma sanguisuga* (Le Conte) and *Triatoma ambigua* neiva as natural carriers of *Trypanosoma cruzi* in Texas. Public Health Rep. 58, 353–354.

Davis, D.J., Sullivan, T., 1946. Complement-fixation test for American trypanosomiasis in Texas. Public Health Rep. 61, 1083–1084.

Deane, M.P., Lenzi, H.L., Jansen, A., 1984. *Trypansoma cruzi*: Vertebrate and invertebrate cycles in the same mammal host, the opossum *Didelphis marsupialis*. Mem. Inst. Osw. Cruz. 79, 513–515.

de la Rua, N., Stevens, L., Dorn, P.L., 2011. High genetic diversity in a single population of *Triatoma sanguisuga* (Le Conte, 1855) inferred from two mitochondrial markers: Cytochrome b and 16S ribosomal DNA. Inf. Genet. Evol. 11, 671–677.

De Shazo, T., 1943. A survey of *Trypanosoma cruzi* infection in Triatoma spp. collected in Texas. J. Bacteriol. 46, 219–220.

Del Castillo, M., Mendoza, G., Oviedo, J., Pérez-Bianco, R.P., Anselmo, A.E., Silva, M., 1990. AIDS and Chagas' disease with central nervos system tumor-like lesion. Am. J. Med. 88, 693–694.

Diamond, L.S., Rubin, R., 1956. Experimental infection of certain farm mammals with North American strain of *Trypanosoma cruzi* from the raccoon. J. Parasitol. 42 (4 Sec. 2), 21.

Diamond, L.S., Rubin, R., 1958. Experimental infection of certain mammals with a North American strain of *Trypanosoma cruzi* from the raccoon. Exp. Parasitol. 7, 383–390.

Dias, E., 1951. Doença de Chagas nas Américas. I. Estados Unidos. Rev. Brasil. Malar. D. Trop. 3, 448–472.

Dias, E., Zeledón, R., 1955. *Infestação domiciliaria* em grau extremo por *Triatoma infestans*. Mem. Inst. Osw. Cruz. 53, 473–486.

Dias, J.C.P., 1968. Manifestações cutâneas na práctica do xenodiagnóstico. Rev. Brasil. Malariol. D. Trop. 20, 248–257.

Di Pentima, M.C., Hwang, L.Y., Skeeter, C.M., Edwards, M.S., 1999. Prevalence of antibody to *Trypanosoma cruzi* in pregnant Hispanic women in Houston. Clin. Inf. Dis. 28, 1281–1285.

Dorn, P.L., Perniciaro, L., Yabsley, M.J., Roelling, D.M., Balsamo, G., Díaz, J., Wesson, D., 2007. Autochthonous transmission of *Trypanosoma cruzi*, Louisiana. Emerg. Infect. Dis. 13, 605–607.

Duprey, Z.H., Steurer, F.J., Rooney, J.A., Kirchhoft, L.V., Jackson, J.E., Rowton, E.D., Schantz, P.M., 2006. Canine visceral leishmaniasis: United States and Canada 2000-2003. Emerg. Inf. Dis. 12, 440–446.

Eads, R.B., Trevino, H.A., Campo, E.G., 1963. Triatoma (Hemiptera: Reduviidae) infected with *Trypanosoma cruzi* in south Texas wood-rat dens. South West Nat. 8, 38–42.

Eberhard, M., D'Alessandro, A., 0027. Congenital *Trypanosoma cruzi* infection in a laboratory-born squirrel monkey, *Saimiri sciureus*. Am. J. Trop. Med. Hyg. 31, 931–933.

Edmiston, W.A., Yokoyama, T., Kay, J., Bilitch, M., Lau, F., 1978. Ventricular tachycardia in a young adult with an apical aneurysm. West. J. Med. 128, 248–253.

Ekkens, D.B., 1981. Nocturnal flights of Triatoma (Hemiptera: Reduviidae) in Sabino Canyon, Arizona. I. Light collections. J. Med. Entomol. 18, 211–227.

Elkins, J.C., 1951a. Chagas disease and vectors in north central Texas. Field Lab. 19, 95–99.

Elkins, J.C., 1951b. The Reduviidae of Texas. Tex. J. Sci. 3, 407–412.

Farrar, W.E., Kagan, I.G., Everton, F.D., Sellers, T.F., 1963. Serologic evidence of human infection with *Trypanosoma cruzi* in Georgia. Am. J. Hyg. 78, 166–172.

Farrar, W.E., Gibbons, S.D., Whitfield, S.T., 1972. Low prevalence of antibody to *Trypanosoma cruzi* in Georgia. Am. J. Trop. Med. Hyg. 21, 404–406.

Feit, S., El-Sherif, N., Korostoff, S., 1983. Chagas' disease masquerading as coronary artery disease. Arch. Inter. Med. 75, 1057–1060.

Fernandes, A.J., Diotaiuti, L., Chiari, E., Dias, J.C.P., 1987. Natural infection of *Didelphys albiventris* by *Trypanosoma cruzi* and *Trypanosoma freitasi*. Mem. Inst. Osw. Cruz. 82 (Suppl. I), 65.

Forattini, O.P., 1980. Biogeografia, origin e distribuição da domililiação de triatomineos no Brasil. Rev. Saude Public 14, 265–299.

Fox, J.C., Ewing, S.A., Buckner, R.G., Whitenack, D., Manley, J.H., 1986. *Trypanosoma cruzi* infection in a dog from Oklahoma. J. Am. Vet. Med. Assoc. 189, 1583–1584.

Galel, S., Kirchhoff, L.V., 1996. Risk factors for *Trypanosoma cruzi* infection in California blood donors. Transfus. 36, 227–231.

Gascon, J., Bern, C., Pinazo, M.J., 2010. Chagas disease in Spain, the United States and other non-endemic countries. Acta Trop. 115, 22–27.

Geiseler, P.J., Ito, J.I., Tegtmeier, B.R., Kerndt, P.R., Krance, R., 1987. Fulminant Chagas disease (CD) in bone marrow transplantation (BMT) (abstract). In: Abstracts of the 1987 Interscience Conference on Antimicrobial Agents and Chemotherapy, New York, October, p. 169.

Gleiser, C.A., Yaeger, R.G., Ghidoni, J.J., 1986. *Trypanosoma cruzi* in a colony-born baboon. J. Am. Vet. Med. Assoc. 189, 1225–1226.

Gluckstein, D., Ciferri, F., Ruskin, J., 1992. Chagas' disease: Another cause of cerebral mass in the acquired immunodeficiency syndrome. Am. J. Med. 92, 429–432.

Goble, F.C., 1958. A comparison of strains of *Trypanosoma cruzi* indigenous to the United States with certain strains from South America. In: Proceedings of 6th International Congress of Tropical Medicine and Malaria 3, 158–166.

Goble, F.C., 1961. Observations on cross- immunity in experimental Chagas disease in dogs. An. Congr. Intl. sôbre D. de Chagas. 2, 602–611.

Goddard, J., 2003. Health problems from "kissing bugs" Infect. Med. (July) 20, 335–338.

Grant, I.H., Gold, J., Wittner, M., Tanowitz, H., Nathan, C., Mayer, K., Reich, L., Wollner, N., Steinherz, L., Ghavimi, F., O'Reilly, R., Armstrong, D., 1989. Transfusion-associated acute Chagas acquired in the United States. Ann. Int. Med. 111, 849–851.

Grögl, M., Kuhn, R.E., Davis, D.S., Green, G.E., 1984. Antibodies to *Trypanosoma cruzi* in coyotes in Texas. J. Parasitol. 70, 189–191.

Grundemann, A.W., 1947. Studies on the biology of *Triatoma sanguisuga* (Le Conte) in Kansas (Reduviidae: Hemiptera). J. Kan. Entomol. Soc. 20, 77–85.

Guzmán-Bracho, C., 2001. Epidemiology of Chagas disease in Mexico: An update. Trends Parasitol. 17, 372–376.

Habermann, R.T., Herman, C.M., Williams, F.P., 1958. Distemper in raccoons and foxes suspected of having rabies. J. Am. Vet. Med. Assoc. 132, 31–35.

Hagar, J.M., Rahimtoola, S.H., 1991. Chagas' heart disease in the United States. N. Engl. J. Med. 325, 763–768.

Hall, C.A., Polizzi, C., Yabsley, M.J., Norton, T.M., 2007. *Trypanosoma cruzi* prevalence and epidemiologic trends in lemurs on St. Catherines Island, Georgia. J. Parasitol. 93, 93–96.

Hancock, K., Zajac, A.M., Pung, O.J., Elvinger, F., Rosypal, A.C., Lindsay, D.S., 2005. Prevalence of antibodies to *Trypanosoma cruzi* in raccoons (*Procyon lotor*) from an urban area of Northern Virginia. J. Parasitol. 91, 470–472.

Hanford, E.J., Zhan, F.B., Lu, Y., Giordano, A., 2007. Chagas disease in Texas: Recognizing the significance and implications of evidence in the literature. Soc. Sc; Med. 65, 60–79.

Hanson, W.L., Derlin, R.F., Roberson, E.L., 1974. Immunoglobulin levels in a laboratory-acquired case of human Chagas' disease. J. Parasitol. 60, 532–533.

Hays, K.L., 1965. Longevity, fecundity and food intake of adult *Triatoma sanguisuga* (Le Conte) Hemiptera: Triatominae. J. Med. Entomol. 2, 200–202.

Hays, K.L., 1966. Some habitat requirements of *Triatoma sanguisuga* (Le Conte) (Hemiptera; Reduviidae). J. Alabama Acad. Sci. 37, 8–14.

Hays, K.L., Turner, H.F., Olsen, P.F., 1961. Chagas' disease in Alabama. Highl. Agric. Res. 8, 4.

Hays, L.H., 1965. The frecuency and magnitude of intraspecific parasitism in *Triatoma sanguisuga* (Le Conte) (Hemiptera). Ecol. 46, 875–877.

Herman, C.M., Bruce Jr., J.I., 1962. Occurrence of *Trypanosoma cruzi* in Maryland. Proc. Helminth. Soc. Wash. 29, 55–58.

Herwaldt, B.L., 2001. Laboratory-acquired parasitic infections from accidental exposures. Clin. Microbiol. Rev. 14, 659–688.

Herwaldt, B.L., Grijalva, M.J., Newsome, A.L., McGhee, C.R., Powell, M.R., Nemec, D.G., Steurer, F.J., Eberhard, M.L., 2000. Use of polymerase chain reaction to diagnose the fifth reported U. S. case of autochtonous transmission of *Trypanosoma cruzi*, in Tennessee, 1998. J. Inf. Dis. 181, 395–399.

Holbert, R.D., Magiros, E., Hirsch, C.P., Nunenmacher, S.J., 1995. Chagas disease: A case in South Mississippi. J. Miss. State Med. Assoc. 36, 1–5.

Houk, A.E., Goodwing, D.G., Zajac, A.M., Barr, S.C., Dubey, J.P., Lindsay, D.S., 2010. Prevalence of antibodies to *Trypanosoma cruzi*, *Toxoplasma gondii*, *Encephalitozoon cuniculi*, *Sarcocystis neurona*, *Besnoitia darlingi* and *Neospora caninum* in North American opossums, *Didelphis virginiana*, from southern Louisiana. J. Parasitol. 96, 1119–1122.

Howard, L.O., 1899. Spider bites and "kissing bugs." Pop. Sci. Mon. 56, 31–42.

Hwang, W.S., Zhang, G., Maslov, D., Weirauch, C., 2010. Short report: Infection rates of *Triatoma protracta* (Uhler) with *Trypanosoma cruzi* in Southern California and molecular identification of trypanosomes. Am. J. Trop. Med. Hyg. 83, 1020–1022.

Ibarra-Cerdeña, C.N., Sánchez-Cordero, V., Peterson, A.T., Ramsey, J.M., 2009. Ecology of North American Triatominae. Acta Trop. 110, 178–186.

Ikenga, J.O., Richerson, J.V., 1984. *Trypanosoma cruzi* (Chagas) (Protozooa: Kinetoplastida: Trypanosomatidae) in invertebrate and vertebrate hosts from Brewster County in Trans-Pecos Texas. J. Econ. Entomol. 77, 126–129.

John, D.T., Hoppe, K.L., 1986. *Trypanosoma cruzi* from wild raccoons in Oklahoma. Am. J. Vet. Res. 47, 1056–1059.

Jurberg, J., Costa, J.M., 1989. Estudos sôbre a resistencia ao jejum e aspectos nutricionais de *Triatoma lecticularia* (Stal, 1859) (Hemiptera, Reduviidae, Triatominae). Mem. Inst. Osw. Cruz 84, 393–399.

Kagan, I.G., Norman, L., Allain, D., 1966. Studies on *Trypanosoma cruzi* isolated in the United States: A rewiew. Rev. Biol. Trop. 14, 55–73.

Karsten, V., Davis, C.R., Kuhn, R., 1992. *Trypanosoma cruzi* in wild raccoons and opossums in North Carolina. J. Parasitol. 78, 547–549.

Kasa, T.J., Lathrop, G.D., Dupuy, H.J., Bonney, C.H., Toft, J.D., 1977. An endemic focus of *Trypanosoma cruzi* infection in a subhuman primate research colony. J. Am. Vet. Med. Assoc. 171, 850–854.

Kerndt, P.R., Wasking, H.A., Kirchhoff, L.V., Steurer, F., Waterman, S.H., Nelson, J.M., Gellert, G.A., Shulman, I.A., 1991. Prevalence of antibody to *Trypanosoma cruzi* among blood donors in Los Angeles, California. Transfus. 31, 814–818.

Kimball, B.M., 1894. *Conorhinus sanguisuga*, its habits and life history. Trans. Kansas Acad. Sc. 14, 128–131.

Kirchhoff, L.V., 1989. Is *Trypanosoma cruzi* a new threat to our blood supply? Ann. Int. Med. 111, 773–775.

Kirchhoff, L.V., 1992. Chagas' disease in non-endemic countries. In: Wendel, S., Brener, Z., Camargo, M.E., Rassi, A. (Eds.), *Chagas' Disease (American Trypanosomiasis): Its Impact on Transfusion and Clinical Medicine*. ISBT Brazil 92, São Paulo, Brazil, pp. 143–152.

Kirchhoff, L.V., 1993. American trypanosomiasis (Chagas' disease): A tropical disease now in the United States. N. Engl. J. Med. 329, 639–644.

Kirchhoff, L.V., Neva, F.A., 1985. American trypanosomiasis (Chagas' disease) in Central American immigrants. JAMA. 254, 3058–3060.

Kirchhoff, L.V., Gam, A.A., Gilliam, F.C., 1987. American trypanosomiasis (Chagas' disease) in Central American immigrants. Am. J. Med. 82, 915–920.

Kitselman, C.H., Grundmann, A.W., 1940. Equine encephalomyelitis virus isolated from naturally infected *Triatoma sanguisuga* (Le Conte). Kansas Agric. Exp. Sta. Tech. Bull. 50, 15.

Kjos, S.A., Snowden, K.F., Craig, T.M., Lewis, B., Ronald, N., Olson, J.K., 2008. Distribution and characterization of canine Chagas disease in Texas. Vet. Parasitol. 152, 249–256.

Kjos, S.A., Snowden, K.F., Olson, J.R., 2009. Biogeography and *Trypanosoma cruzi* infection prevalence of Chagas disease vectors in Texas, USA. Vector-Borne Zoonot. Dis. 9, 41–50.

Klotz, J.H., Dorn, P.L., Logan, J.L., Stevens, L., Pinnas, J.L., Schmidt, J.O., Klotz, S.A., 2010. Kissing bugs: Potential disease vectors and cause of anaphylaxis. Clin. Infect. Dis. 50, 1629–1634.

Klotz, S.A., Dorn, P.L., Klotz, J.H., Pinnas, J.L., Weirauch, C., Kurtz, J.R., Schmidt, J., 2009. Feeding behavior of triatomines from the southwestern United States: An update on potential risk for transmission of Chagas disease. Acta Trop. 111, 114–118.

Kofoid, C.A., McCulloch, I., 1916. On *Trypanosoma triatomae*, a new flagellate from a hemipteran bug from the nests of the wood rat, *Neotoma fuscipes*. Univ. Calif. Public Zool. 16, 113–126 and pl 14–15.

Kofoid, C.A., Donat, F., 1933a. Experimental infection with *Trypanosoma cruzi* from intestine of cone-nose bug, *Triatoma protracta*. Proc. Soc. Exp. Biol. Med. 30, 489–491.

Kofoid, C.A., Donat, F., 1933b. South American trypanosomiasis of the human type – Occurrence in mammals in the United States. Calif. West. Med. 38, 245.

Kofoid, C.A., Wood, F.D., McNeil, E., 1935. The cycle of *Trypanosoma cruzi* in tissue cultures of embryonic heart muscle. Univ. Calif. Public Zool. 41, 23–24.

Kofoid, C.A., Whitaker, B.G., 1936. Natural infection of American human trypanosomiasis in two species of cone-nosed bugs, *Triatoma protracta* Uhler and *Triatoma uhleri* Neiva, in the Western United States. J. Parasitol. 22, 259–263.

Kofoid, C.A., McNeil, E., Wood, F.D., 1937. Effects of arsenicals on *Trypanosoma cruzi* in tissue cultures. J. Pharmacol. Exp. Ther. 59, 424–428.

Kun, H., Moore, A., Mascola, L., Steurer, F., Gena, I., Kubak, B., Radhakrishna, S., Leiby, D., Herron, R., Mone, T., Hunter, R., Kurhnert, M., 2009. Transmission of *Trypanosoma cruzi* by heart transplantation. Clin. Inf. Dis. 48, 1534–1540.

Lambert, R.C., Kolivras, K.N., Resler, L.M., Brewster, C.C., Paulson, S.L., 2008. The potential for emergence of Chagas disease in the United States. Geospat. Health 2, 227–239.

Lane, D.J., Sher, G., Ward, B., Ndao, M., Leiby, D.A., Hewlett, B., Bow, E., 2000. Investigation on the second case of transfusion-transmitted Chagas disease in Canada. Blood 96, 60a (Abstract 252).

Lapierre, J., Lariviere, M., 1954. Reaction allergigue aux picures de reduvidés (*Rhodnius prolixus*). Bull. Soc. Path. Ex. 4, 563–566.

Lathrop, G.D., Ominsky, A.J., 1965. Chagas' disease study in a group of individuals bitten by North American triatomids. USAF School of Aerospace Medicine, Aerospace Medical Division (AFSC), Brooks Air Force Base, Texas, Review 9–65, 5.

Le Conte, J., 1855. Remarks on two species of American Cimex. Proc. Acad. Nat. Sc. Philadelphia. 7, 404.

Leiby, D.A., Read, E.J., Lenes, B.A., Yund, A.J., Stumpf, R.J., Kirchhoff, L.V., Dodd, R.Y., 1997. Seroepidemiology of *Trypanosoma cruzi* etiologic agent of Chagas' disease in U.S. blood donors. J. Infect. Dis. 176, 1047–1052.

Leiby, D.A., Fucci, M.H., Stumpf, R.J., 1999. *Trypanosoma cruzi* in a low-to moderate-risk blood donor population: Seroprevalence and possible congenital transmission. Transfus. 39, 310–317.

Leiby, D.A., Lener, B.A., Tibbals, M.A., Tames-Olmedo, M.T., 1999. Prospective evaluation of a patient with *Trypanosoma cruzi* infection transmitted by transfusion. New Engl. J. Med. 341, 1237–1238.

Leiby, D.A., Rentas, F.J., Nelson, K.E., Stambolis, V.A., Ness, P.M., Parnis, C., McAllister, H.A., Yawn, D.H., Stumpf, R.J., Kirchhoff, L.V., 2000. Evidence of *Trypanosoma cruzi* infection (Chagas disease) among patients undergoing cardiac surgery. Circ. 102, 2978–2982.

Leiby, D.A., Herron, R.M., Read, E.J., Lenes, B.A., Stumpf, R.J., 2002. *Trypanosoma cruzi* in Los Angeles and Miami blood donors: Impact of evolving donor demographics on seroprevalence and implications for transfusion transmission. Transfus. 42, 549–555.

Leiby, D.A., 2004. Threats to blood safety posed by emerging protozoan pathogens. Vox Sang. 87 (Suppl. 2), S120–S122.

Lent, H., Wygodzinsky, P., 1979. Revision of the Triatominae (Reduviidae, Hemiptera) and their significance as vector of Chagas' disease. Bull. Am. Mus. Nat. Hist. 163, 125–520.

Lent, H., Jurgerg, J., 1987. A genitalia externa dos machos de sete especies de Triatoma Laporte, 1832 da Região Neártica (Hemiptera, Reduviidae, Triatominae). Mem. Inst. Osw. Cruz. 82, 227–246.

Lesser, E., Lukeman, J.M., 1957. Stomach infections with *Trypanosoma cruzi*. J. Parasitol. 43, 65.

Libow, L.F., Beltrani, V.P., Silvers, D.N., Grossman, M.E., 1991. Post-cardiac transplant reactivation of Chagas' disease diagnosed by skin biopsy. Cutis. 48, 37–40.

Lorenzana, R., 1967. Chronic Chagas' myocarditis: Report of a case. Am. J. Clin. Pathol. 48, 39–43.

Lynch, P.J., Pinnas, J.L., 1978. "Kissing bug" bites: Triatoma species as an important cause of insect bites in the southwest. Cutis. 22, 585–589.

Maekelt, G.A., 1974. Discussion. In: Trypanosomiasis and Leishmaniasis with special reference to Chagas disease. Ciba Foundation Symposium 20 (New Series), Elsevier, Excerpta Medica, p. 80.

Marlatt, C.L., 1896. The bed bug and cone-nose. U. S. Div. Entomol. N. S. Bull. 4, 32–42.

Marshall, N.A., Street, D.H., 1982. Allergy to *Triatoma protracta* (Heteroptera: Reduviidae). I. Etiology, antigen preparation, diagnosis and immunotherapy. J. Med. Entomol. 19, 248–252.

Marshall, N.A., Liebhaber, M., Dyer, Z., Saxon, A., 1986. The prevalence of allergic sensitization to *Triatoma protracta* (Heteroptera: Reduviidae) in a southern California, USA, community. J. Med. Entomol. 23, 117–124.

Martínez-Ibarra, J.A., Galavis-Silva, L., Lara-Campos, C., Trujillo-García, J.C., 1992. Distribución de los triatominos asociados al domicilio humano en el municipio de general Terán, Nuevo León, México. Southwest Entomol. 17, 261–265.

Martínez-Ibarra, J.A., Nogueda-Torres, B., Paredes-González, E., Alexandre-Aguilar, R., Solorio-Cibrián, M., Barreto, S.P., Gómez-Estrada, H.I., Trujillo-García, J.C., 2005. Development of Triatoma rubida sonoriana, Triatoma barberi and Meccus mazzottii (Heteroptera, Reduviidae) under laboratory conditions. J. Am. Mosq. Contr. Assoc. 21, 310–315.

Martínez-Ibarra, J.A., Alejandre-Aguilar, R., Paredes-González, E., Martínez-Silva, M.A., Solario-Cibrián, M., Nogueda-Torres, B., Trujillo-Contreras, F., Novelo-López, M., 2007. Biology of three species of North American Triatominae (Hemiptera: Reduviidae: Triatominae) fed on rabbits. Mem. Inst. Osw. Cruz. 102, 925–930.

Martins, A.V., 1968. Epidemiologia da Doença de Chagas. In: Cançado, J.R. (Ed.), Doença de Chagas. Belo Horizonte, Imprensa Oficial, pp. 225–237.

Mascola, L., Kubak, B., Radhakrishna, S., Mone, T., Hunter, R., Leiby, DA., Kuehnert, M., Moore, A., Steurer, F., Lawrence, G., Kun, H., 2006. Chagas disease alter organ transplantation, Los Angeles, California, CDC. MMWR. Morb. Mortal. Wkly. Rep. 55, 798–799.

Massumi, R.A., Gooch, A., 1965. Chagas' myocarditis. Arch. Inter. Med. 116, 531–536.

McKeever, S., Gorman, G.W., Norman, L., 1958. Occurrence of a Trypanosoma cruzi-like organism in some mammals from southwestern Georgia and northwestern Florida. J. Parasitol. 44, 583–587.

Mehringer, P.J., Wood, S.F., 1958. A resampling of wood rat house and human habitations in Griffith Park, Los Angeles, for Triatoma protracta and Trypanosoma cruzi. Bull. South Calif. Acad. Sc. 57, 39–46.

Mehringer, P.J., Wood, S.F., Anderson, R.C., 1961. Cone nose bug (Triatoma) annoyance and Trypanosoma cruzi in Griffith Park in 1960. Bull. South Calif. Acad. Sci. 60, 190–192.

Metze, K., Maciel, J.A., 1993. AIDS and Chagas' disease. Neurol. 43, 447–448.

Meurs, K.M., Anthony, M.A., Slater, M., Miller, M.V., 1998. Chronic Trypanosoma cruzi infection in dogs: 11 cases (1987–1996). J. Am. Vet. Med. Assoc. 213, 497–500.

Milei, J., Mantner, B., Storino, R., Sánchez, J.A., Ferranz, V.J., 1992. Does Chagas' disease exist as an underdiagnosed form of cardiomyopathy in the United States? Am. Heart J. 123, 1732–1735.

Moffitt, J.E., Venarske, D., Goddard, J., Yates, A.B., de Shazo, R.D., 2003. Allergic reactions to Triatoma bites. Ann. Allergy Asthma Immunol. 91, 122–128.

Moncayo, A., Ortiz-Yanine, M.I., 2006. An update on Chagas disease (human American trypanosomiasis). Ann. Trop. Med. Parasitol. 100, 663–677.

Montalvo-Hicks, L.D.C., Trevenen, C.L., Briggs, J.N., 1980. American trypanosomiasis (Chagas' disease) in a Canadian immigrant infant. Pediatrics. 66, 266–268.

Morrill, A.W., 1914. Some American insects and arachnids concerned in the transmission of disease. Arizona Med. J. 2, 14–25.

Mortensen, F.W., Walsh, J.D., 1963. Review of the Triatoma protracta problem in the Sierra Nevada foothills of California. Proceedings and Papers of 31st Annual Conference of the California Mosquito Control Association pp. 44–45.

Mott, K.E., França, J.T., Barrett, T.V., Hoff, R., de Oliveira, T.S., Sherlock, I.A., 1980. Cutaneous allergic reactions to Triatoma infestans after xenodiagnosis. Mem. Inst. Osw. Cruz. 75, 3–10.

Nabity, M.B., Barnhart, K., Logan, K.S., Santos, R.L., Kessell, A., Melmed, C., Snowden, K.F., 2006. An atypical case of Trypanosoma cruzi infection in a young English Mastiff. Vet. Parasitol. 140, 356–361.

Nascimento, R.J., Santana, J.M., Lozzi, S.P., Araújo, C.N., Teixeira, A.R.L., 2001. Human IgG$_1$ and IgG$_4$: The main antibodies against Triatoma infestans (Hemiptera: Reduviidae) salivary gland proteins. Am. J. Trop. Med. Hyg. 65, 219–226.

Navin, T.R., Roberto, R.R., Juranek, D.D., Limpakarnjanarat, K., Mortenson, E.W., Clover, J.R., Yescott, R.E., Taclindo, C., Steurer, F., Allain, D., 1985. Human and sylvatic *Trypanosoma cruzi* infection in California. Am. J. Public Health 75, 366–369.

Neiva, A., 1911. Notas de entomologia medica. Duas novas especies norte-americanas de hemipteros hematofagos. Brasil Med. 25, 421–422.

Neiva, A., 1914. *Revisão do gênero Triatoma Lap.* Tese, Faculdade de Medicina. Rio de Janeiro, Brazil. p. 80.

Neiva, A., Lent, H., 1941. Sinopse dos Triatomideos. Rev. Entomol. 12, 61–92.

Nichols, N., Green, T.W., 1963. Allergic reactions to "kissing bugs" bites. Calif. Med. 98, 267–268.

Nickerson, P., Orr, P., Schroeder, M.L., Sekla, L., Johnston, J.B., 1989. Transfusion-associated *Trypanosoma cruzi* infection in a non-endemic area. Ann. Int. Med. 111, 851–853.

Nieto, P.D., Boushton, R., Dorn, P.L., Steurer, F., Raychandhuri, S., Esfandiari, J., Gonçalves, E., Díaz, J., Malone, J.B., 2009. Comparison of two immunochromatographic assays and the indirect immunoflorescence antibody test for diagnosis of *Trypansoma cruzi* infection in dogs in south central Louisiana. Vet. Parasitol. 65, 241–247.

Nissen, E.E., Roberson, E.L., Lipham, L.B., Hanson, W.L., 1977. Naturally occurring Chagas' disease in a South Carolina puppy. 114th Annual AVMA Meeting of the American Association of Veterinary Parasitologists, Atlanta, GA.

Nogueda-Torres, B., Alejandre-Aguilar, R., Isita-Tornell, L., Camacho, A.D., 2000. Defaecation patterns in seven species of triatomines (Insecta, Reduviidae) present in Mexico. Rev. Latinoam. Microbiol. 42, 145–148.

Norman, L., Brooke, M.M., Allain, D.S., Gorman, G.W., 1959. Morphology and virulence of *Trypanosoma cruzi*-like hemoflagellates isolated from wild mammals in Georgia and Florida. J. Parasitol. 45, 457–463.

Nowicki, M.J., Chinchilla, C., Corado, L., Matsuoka, L., Selby, R., Steurer, F., Mone, T., Méndez, R., Aswad, S., 2006. Prevalence of antibodies to *Trypanosoma cruzi* among solid organ donors in southern California: A population at risk. Transplant. 81, 477–479.

Ochs, D.E., Hnilica, V.S., Moser, D.R., Smith, J.H., Kirchhoff, L.V., 1996. Post mortem diagnosis of autochtonous acute Chagas myocarditis by polymerase chain reaction amplification of a species-specific DNA sequence of *Trypanosoma cruzi*. Am. J. Trop. Med. Hyg. 54, 526–529.

Olsen, P.F., Schoemaker, J.P., Turner, H.F., Hays, K.L., 1964. Incidence of *Trypanosoma cruzi* (Chagas) in wild vectors and reservoirs in East- Central Alabama. J. Parasitol. 50, 599–603.

Olson, L.C., Skinner, S.F., Patolay, J.L., McGhee, G.E., 1986. Encephalitis associated with *Trypanosoma cruzi* in a celebes black macaque. Lab. Anim. Sci. 36, 667–670.

OPS. 2011. Iniciativa de los Países de América Central para la Interrupción de la Transmisión Vectorial y Transfusional de la Enfermedad de Chagas (IPCA). Historia de 12 años de una Iniciativa Subregional 1998-2010, Tegucigalpa, Honduras, p. 89.

Packchanian, A., 1939. Natural infection of *Triatoma gerstaeckeri* with *Trypanosoma cruzi* in Texas. Public Health Rep. 54, 1547–1554.

Packchanian, A., 1940a. Natural infection of *Triatoma heidemanni* with *Trypanosoma cruzi* in Texas. Public Health Rep. 55, 1300–1306.

Packchanian, A., 1940b. Experimental transmission of *Trypanosoma cruzi* infection in animals by *Triatoma sanguisuga ambigua*. Public Health Rep. 55, 1526–1532.

Packchanian, A., 1942. Reservoir hosts of Chagas disease in the state of Texas. Natural infection of nine-banded armadillos (*Dasypus novemcinctus texanus*), house mice (*Mus musculus*), opossum (*Didelphis virginiana*) and wood rats (*Neotoma micropus micropus*), with *Trypanosoma cruzi* in the state of Texas. Am. J. Trop. Med. 22, 623–631.

Packchanian, A., 1943. Infectivity of the Texas strain of *Trypanosoma cruzi* to man. Am. J. Trop. Med. 23, 309–314.

Packchanian, A., 1947. The problem of Chagas' disease in the state of Texas. Texas Med. 43, 179–183.

Packchanian, A., 1949. The present status of Chagas' disease in the United States. Rev. Soc. Mex. Hist. Nat. 10, 91–101.

Paddock, C.D., McKerrow, J.H., Hansell, E., Foreman, K.W., Hsieh, I., Marshall, N., 2001. Identification, cloning and recombinant expression of Procalin, a major Triatomine allergen. J. Immunol. 167, 2694–2699.

Paige, C.F., Scholl, D.T., Truman, R.W., 2002. Prevalence and incidence density of *Mycobacterium leprae* and *Trypanosoma cruzi* infection within a population of wild nine-banded armadillos. Am. J. Trop. Med. Hyg. 67, 528–532.

Paredes, G.E.A., Valdez-Miranda, J., Nogueda-Torres, B., Alejandre-Aguilar, R., Canett-Romero, R., 2001. Vectorial importance of Triatominae bugs (Hemiptera: Reduviidae) in Guaymas. Mexico. Rev. Latinoam. Microbiol. 43, 119–122.

Pearlman, J.D., 1983. Chagas' disease in Northern California. No longer an endemic diagnosis. Am. J. Med. 75, 1057–1060.

Pereira, M.H., Souza, M.E.L., Vargas, A.P., Martins, M.S., Penido, C.M., Diotaiuti, L., 1996. Anticoagulant activity of *Triatoma infestans* and *Panstrongylus megistus* saliva (Hemiptera/Triatominae). Acta Trop. 61, 255–261.

Peterson, A.T., Sánchez-Cordero, V., Beard, C.B., Ramsey, J.M., 2002. Ecologic niche modeling and potential reservoirs for Chagas disease. Mexico. Emerg. Infect. Dis. 8, 662–667.

Pfeiler, E., Bitter, B.G., Ramsey, J.M., Palacios-Cardiel, C., Markow, T.A., 2006. Genetic variation, population structure and phylogenetic relationships of *Triatoma rubida* and *T. recurva* (Hemiptera: Reduviidae: Triatominae) from the Sonoran desert, insect vectors of Chagas disease parasite *Trypanosoma cruzi*. Mol. Phylogenet. Evol. 41, 209–221.

Pietrzak, S.M., Pung, O.J., 1998. Trypanosomiasis in raccoons from Georgia. J. Wild. Dis. 34, 132–136.

Pinnas, J.L., Chen, T.M.W., Hoffman, D.R., 1978. Evidence for IgE mediation of human sensitivity to Reduviid bug bites. Fed. Proc. 37, 1555.

Pinnas, J.L., Lindberg, R.E., Chen, T.M.W., Meinke, G.C., 1986. Studies of kissing bug-sensitive patients: Evidence for the lack of cross-reactivity between *Triatoma protracta* and *Triatoma rubida* salivary gland extract. J. Allergy Clin. Immunol. 77, 364–370.

Pippin, W.F., Law, P.F., Gaylor, M.J., 1968. *Triatoma sanguisuga* texana Usinger and *Triatoma sanguisuga* indictiva Neiva naturally infected with *Trypanosoma cruzi* Chagas in Texas. J. Med. Entomol. 5, 134.

Pippin, W.F., 1970. The biology and vector capability of *Triatoma sanguisuga texana usinger* and *Triatoma gerstaeckeri* (Stål) compared with *Rhodnius prolixus* (Stål) (Hemiptera: Triatominae). J. Med. Entomol. 7, 30–45.

Porter, J.A., 1965. *Triatoma sanguisuga* (Le Conte, 1855) in Illinois. J. Parasitol. 51, 500.

Pung, O.J., Banks, C.W., Jones, D.N., Krissinger, M.W., 1995. *Trypanosoma cruzi* in wild raccoons, opossums and triatomine bugs in Southeast Georgia, U.S.A. J. Parasitol. 81, 324–326.

Pung, O.J., Spratt, J., Graham, C., Norton, T.M., Carter, J., 1998. *Trypanosoma cruzi* infection of free-ranging lion-tailed macaques (*Macaca silenus*) and ring-tailed lemurs (*Lemur catta*) on St. Catherine's Island, Georgia, USA. J. Zoo. Wild. Med. 29, 25–30.

Readio, P.A., 1927. Studies on the biology of the Reduviidae of America north of Mexico. Kans. Univ. Sci. Bull. 17, 5–241.

Reinhard, K., Fink, T.M., Skiles, J., 2003. A case of megacolon in Rio Grande Valley as a possible case of Chagas' disease. Mem. Inst. Osw. Cruz. 98 (Suppl. I), 165–172.

Reisenman, C.E., Lawrence, G., Guerenstein, T.G., Dotson, H., Hildebrand, J.G., 2010. Infection of kissing bugs with *Trypanosoma cruzi*, Tucson, Arizona, USA. Emerg. Inf. Dis. 16, 400–405.

Ribeiro, J.M.C., Schneider, M., Isaías, T., Jurberg, J., Galvão, C., Guimarães, J.A., 1998. Role of salivary antihemostatic components in blood feeding by triatomine bugs (Heteroptera). J. Med. Entomol. 35, 599–609.

Rocha, D.S., Jurberg, J., Galvão, C., 1996. Descrição dos ovos o ninfas de *Triatoma lecticularia* (Stål, 1859) (Hemiptera, Reduviidae, Triatominae). Entomol. Vect. 3, 123–135.

Roelling, D.M., Brown, E.L., Barnabe, C., Tibayrenc, M., Steurer, F.J., Yabsley, M.J., 2008. Molecular typing of *Trypanosoma cruzi* isolates, United States. Emerg. Inf. Dis. 14, 1123–1125.

Roelling, D.M., Ellis, A.E., Yasbley, M.J., 2009. Genetically different isolates of *Trypanosoma cruzi* elicit different infection dynamics in raccoons (*Procyon lotor*) and Virginia opossums (*Didelphis virginiana*). Int. J. Parasitol. 39, 1603–1610.

Rohr, A.S., Marshall, N.A., Saxon, A., 1984. Successful immunotherapy for *Triatoma protracta*-induced anaphylaxis. J. Allergy Clin. Immunol. 73, 369–375.

Rosypal, A.C., Tidwell, R.R., Lindsay, D.S., 2007. Prevalence of antibodies to *Leishmania infantum* and *Trypansoma cruzi* in wild canids from South Carolina. J. Parasitol. 93, 955–957.

Rosypal, A.C., Tripp, S., Francis, J., Stoskopf, M.K., Larsen, R.S., Lindsay, D.S., 2010. Survey of antibodies to *Trypanosoma cruzi* and *Leishmania spp.* in gray and red fox populations from North Carolina and Virginia. J. Parasitol. 96, 1230–1231.

Ryan, C.P., Hughes, P.E., Howard, E.B., 1985. American trypanosomiasis (Chagas' disease) in a striped skunk. J. Wildl. Dis. 21, 175–176.

Ryckman, R.E., 1951. Recent observations of cannibalism in Triatoma (Hemiptera: Reduviidae). J. Parasitol. 37, 433–434.

Ryckman, R.E., 1953. First report of *Paratriatoma hirsuta* Barber from Nevada and additional collections from Arizona and California. Pan-Pacific Entomol. 29, 199.

Ryckman, R.E., 1962. Biosystematics and hosts of the *Triatoma protracta* complex in North America. Univ. Calif. Public Entomol. 27, 93–249 and pl. 24.

Ryckman, R.E., 1967. Six new populations of Triatominae from western North America (Hemiptera; Reduviidae). Bull. Pan-Am. Res. Inst. 1, 1–3.

Ryckman, R.E., 1971. The genus *Paratriatoma* in western North America (Hemiptera: Reduviidae). J. Med. Entomol. 8, 87–97.

Ryckman, R.E., 1979. Host reactions to bug bites (Hemiptera: Homoptera): A literature review and annotated bibliography, Part I. Calif. Vec. Views 26, 1–24.

Ryckman, R.E., 1981. The kissing bug problem in western North America. Bull. Soc. Vec. Ecol. 6, 167–169.

Ryckman, R.E., 1984. The Triatominae of North and Central America and the West Indies: A checklist with synonymy (Hemiptera: Reduviidae: Triatominae). Bull. Soc. Vec. Ecol. 9, 71–83.

Ryckman, R.E., 1985. Dermatological reactions to the bites of four species of Triatominae (Hemiptera: Reduviidae) and *Cimex lectularius* (Hemiptera: Cimicidae). Bull. Soc. Vec. Ecol. 10, 122–125.

Ryckman, R.E., 1986. The vertebrate hosts of the Triatominae of North and Central America and the West Indies (Hemiptera: Reduviidae: Triatominae). Bull. Soc. Vec. Ecol. 11, 221–241.

Ryckman, R.E., Folkes, D.L., Olsen, L.E., Robb, P.L., Ryckman, A.E., 1965. Epizootiology of *Trypanosoma cruzi* in southwestern North America. J. Med. Entomol. 2, 87–108.

Ryckman, R.E., Ryckman, J.V., 1967. Epizootiology of *Trypanosoma cruzi* in southwestern North America. Part XII: Does Gause's rule apply to ectoparasitic Triatominae? (Hemiptera: Reduviidae) (Kinetoplastidae: Trypanosomidae) (Rodentia: Cricetidae). J. Med. Entomol. 4, 379–386.

Ryckman, R.E., Casdin, M.A., 1976. The Triatominae of western North America, a checklist and bibliography. Calif. Vec. Views. 23, 35–52.

Ryckman, R.E., Bentley, D.G., 1979. Host reactions to bug bites (Hemiptera, Homoptera): A literature review and annotated bibliography. Part II. Calif. Vec. Views. 26, 25–49.

Ryley, C.V., Howard, L.O., 1892. Notes on the "blood-sucking cone-nose." Insect Life 4, 273–274.

Ryley, C.V., Howard, L.O., 1893. On the habits of the "variegated cone-nose." Insect Life 5, 203–204.

Ryley, C.V., Howard, L.O., 1894. The blood-sucking cone-nose again. Insect Life 6, 267.

Sandoval, C.M., Gutiérrez, R., Luna, S., Amaya, M., Esteban, L., Ariza, H., Angulo, V.M., 2000. High density of *Rhodnius prolixus* in a rural house in Colombia. Trans. Roy. Soc. Trop. Med. Hyg. 94, 372–373.

Saulnier Sholler, G.L., Kalkunte, S., Greenlaw, C., McCarten, K., Forman, E., 2006. Antitumor activity of nifurtimox observed in a patient with neuroblastoma. J. Pediatr. Hematol. Oncol. 28, 693–695.

Schaffer, G.D., Hanson, W.L., Davidson, W.R., Nettles, F., 1978. Hematotropic parasites of translocated raccoons in the southeast. J. Am. Vet. Med. Assoc. 173, 1148–1151.

Scherb, J., Arias, I.M., 1962. Achalasia of the esophagus and Chagas' disease. Gastroenterol. 43, 212–215.

Schielke, J.E., Selvarangan, R., Kyes, K.B., Fritsche, T.R., 2002. Laboratory diagnosis of *Trypanosoma cruzi* infection in a colony-raised pigtail macaque. Contemp. Top. Lab. Anim. Sci. 41, 42–45.

Schiffler, R.J., Mansur, G.P., Navin, T.R., Limpakarnjanarat, K., 1984. Indigenous Chagas' disease (American Trypanosomiasis) in California. J. Am. Med. Assoc. 251, 2983–2984.

Schmuñis, G.A., 1991. *Trypanosoma cruzi*, the etiologic agent of Chagas' disease: Status in the blood supply in endemic and non-endemic countries. Transfus. 31, 547–557.

Schofield, C.J., Jannin, J., Salvatella, R., 2006. The future of Chagas disease control. Trends Parasitol. 22, 583–588.

Schuck, B.R., 1945. A new locality for *Trypanosoma cruzi* in Arizona. J. Parasitol. 31, 151.

Seibold, H.R., Wolf, R.H., 1970. American trypanosomiasis (Chagas' disease) in Hylobates pileatus. Lab. Anim. Care. 20, 514–517.

Shadomy, S.V., Waring, S.C., Martins-Filho, O.A., Oliveira, R.C., Chapell, C.L., 2004. Combined use of enzyme-linked immunosorbent assay and flow cytometry to detect antibodies to *Trypanosoma cruzi* in domestic canines in Texas. Clin. Diag. Lab. Immunol. 11, 313–319.

Shafi, A., 1977. Chagas' disease with cardiopathy and hemiplegia. N. Y. State J. Med. 77, 418–419.

Shields, T.L., Walsh, E.M., 1956. "Kissing bug" bite. Arch. Dermatol. 74, 14–21.

Shulman, L.A., Appleman, S.S., Hiti, A.L., Kirchhoff, L.V., 1997. Specific antibodies to *Trypanosoma cruzi* among blood donors in Los Angeles. California. Transfus. 37, 727–731.

Sjögren, R.D., Ryckman, R.E., 1966. Epizootiology of *Trypanosoma cruzi* in southwestern North America. Part VIII: Nocturnal flights of *Triatoma protracta* (Uhler) as indicated by collection at black light traps (Hemiptera: Reduviidae: Triatominae). J. Med. Entomol. 3, 81–92.

Skolnick, A., 1989. Does influx from endemic areas mean more transfusion-associated Chagas' disease? JAMA. 262, 1443.

Skolnick, A., 1991. Deferral aims to deter Chagas' parasite. JAMA. 265, 173.

Snider, T.G., Yaeger, R.G., Dellucky, J., 1980. Myocarditis caused by *Trypanosoma cruzi* in a native Louisiana dog. J. Am. Vet. Med. Assoc. 177, 247–249.

Stål, C., 1859. Monographie der Gattung Conorhinus und Verwandten. Berl. Entomol. Zeitschr. 3, 99–117.

Steindel, M., Scholz, A.F., Toma, H.K., Carvalho Pinto, J.C., Schlemper Jr., B.R., 1987. Parasitism of blood and anal glands of naturally infected opossum (*Didelphis marsupialis*) from the Arvoredo Island, Santa Catarina by *Trypansoma cruzi*. Mem. Inst. Osw. Cruz. 82 (Suppl. I), 66.

Stolf, N.A., Higushi, L., Bocchi, E., Bellotti, G., Auler, J.O.C., Uip, D., Neto, V.A., Pileggi, F., Jatene, D., 1987. Heart transplantation in patients with Chagas' disease cardiomyopathy. J. Heart Transplant. 6, 307–312.

Stramer, S.L., Dadd, R.Y., Leiby, D.A. et al., 2007. Blood donor screening for Chagas disease – United States, 2006–2007. MMWR. 56, 141–143.

Sullivan, T.D., McGregor, T., Eads, R.B., Davis, D.J., 1949. Incidence of *Trypanosoma cruzi* Chagas in Triatoma (Hemiptera: Reduviidae) in Texas. Am. J. Trop. Med. Hyg. 29, 453–458.

Swezey, R.L., 1963. "Kissing bug" bite in Los Angeles. Arch. Inter. Med. 112, 977–980.

Tanowitz, H.B., Kirchhoff, L.V., Simon, D., Morris, S.A., Weiss, L.M., Wittner, M., 1992. Chagas' disease. Clin. Microbiol. Rev. 5, 400–419.

Tanowitz, H.B., Weiss, L.M., Montgomery, S.P., 2011. Chagas disease has now gone global. PLoS Negl. Trop. Dis. 5, e1136.

Telford, S.R., Forrester, D.J., 1991. Hemoparasites of raccoons (*Procyon lotor*) in Florida. J. Wildl. Dis. 27, 486–490.

Teo, S.K., Cheah, J.S., 1973. Severe reactions to the bite of the triatomid bug (*Triatoma rubrofasciata*) in Singapore. J. Trop. Med. Hyg. 76, 161–162.

Thurman, D.C., 1944. The biology of *Triatoma neotomae* Neiva in Texas. J. Econom. Entomol. 37, 116–117.

Thurman, D.C., 1945a. The biology of *Triatoma gerstaeckeri*. J. Econ. Entomol. 38, 597–598.

Thurman, D.C., 1945b. The blood sucking habits and growth of nymphs of *Triatoma gerstaeckeri*. J. Econ. Entomol. 38, 597.

Thurman, D.C., Mulrennan, J.A., Basham, E., Taylor, D.J., 1948. Key to Florida Triatoma with additional distribution records for the species. Florida Entomol. 31, 58–62.

Tippit, T.S., 1978. *Canine trypanosomiasis* (Chagas' disease). Southwest Vet. 31, 97–104.

Tobler, L.H., Contestable, P., Pitina, L., Groth, H., Shafer, S., Blackburn, G.R., Warren, H., Lee, S.R., Busch, M.P., 2007. Evaluation of a new enzyme linked immunosorbent assay for detection of Chagas antibody in US donors. Transfus. 47, 90–96.

Tomlinson, M.J., Chapman, W.L., Hanson, W.L., Gosser, H.S., 1981. Occurrence of anti-body to *Trypanosoma cruzi* in dogs in the southeastern United States. Am. J. Vet. Res. 42, 1444–1446.

Tonn, R.J., 1985. Estados Unidos. In: Carcavallo, R.U., Rabinovich, J. E., Tonn, R.J. (Eds.), *Factores Biológicos y Ecológicos en la Enfermedad de Chagas*. Centro Panamericano de Ecología Humana y Salud, Argentina, 2, 429–436.

Uhler, P.R., 1876. List of Hemiptera of the region west of the Mississippi River, including those collected during the Hayden Exploration of 1873. Bull. U.S. Geol., Geogr. Surv. Terr. 5 (2nd series), 267–361.

Uhler, P.R., 1878. Notices of the Hemiptera Heteroptera in the collection of the late T. W. Harris, M.D. Proc. Boston Soc. Nat. Hist. 19, 365–446.

Usinger, R.L., 1939. Description of new Triatominae with a key to genera (Hemiptera, Reduviidae). Univ. Calif. Public Entomol. 7, 33–56.

Usinger, R.L., 1944. The Triatominae of North and Central America. Public Health Bull. 288, 81.

Usinger, R.L., Wigodzinsky, P., Ryckman, R.E., 1966. The biosystematics of Triatominae. Ann. Rev. Entomol. 11, 309–330.

Vakalis, N., Miller, J.H., Lauritsen, E., Hansen, D., 1983. Anti-*Trypanosoma cruzi* antibodies among domestic dogs in New Orleans. J. La State Med. Soc. 135, 14–15.

Verani, J.R., Montgomery, S.P., Schulkin, J., Anderson, B., Jones, J.L., 2010. Survey of obstetrician-gynecologists in the United States about Chagas disease. Am. J. Trop. Med. Hyg. 83, 891–895.

Walsh, B.D., Riley, C.V., 1869. The blood-sucking cone-nose, or big bedbug. Am. Entomol. 1, 87–88.

Walsh, J.D., Jones, J.P., 1962. Public health significance of the cone-nosed bug, *Triatoma protracta* (Uhler) in the Sierra Nevada foothills of California. Calif. Vec. Views. 9, 33–36.

Walton, B.C., Bauman, P.M., Diamond, L.S., Herman, C.M., 1956. *Trypanosoma cruzi* in raccoons from Maryland. J. Parasitol. 42 (Suppl.), 20.

Walton, B.C., Bauman, P.M., Diamond, L.S., Herman, C.M., 1958. The isolation and identification of *Trypanosoma cruzi* from raccoons in Maryland. Am. J. Trop. Med. Hyg. 7, 603–610.

Wehrle, L.P., 1939. Observations on three species of Triatoma (Hemiptera: Reduviidae). Bull. Brooklyn Entomol. Soc. 34, 145–154.

Western, K.A., Schultz, M.G., Farrar, W.E., Kagan, I.G., 1969. Laboratory-acquired Chagas' disease treated with Bay 2502. Bol. Chileno Parasitol. 24, 94.

Whittacker, F.H., Jarecha, L., 1974. An examination of opossums and raccoons in Kentucky for natural infections with *Trypanosoma cruzi*. Trans. Kentucky Acad. Sc. 35, 76–78.

WHO. 1991. Control of Chagas disease. Report of a WHO Expert Committee, WHO Technical Report Series 811, p. 95.

WHO. 1995 Tropical disease research: Progress 1975-94: Highlights 1993–94. Twelfth Programme Report of the UNDP/World Bank/WHO Special Programme for Research and Training in Tropical Diseases (TDR), p. 167.

Williams, G.D., Adams, L.G., Yaeger, R.G., McGrath, R.K., Read, W.K., Bilderback, W.R., 1977. Naturally occurring trypanosomiasis (Chagas' disease) in dogs. J. Am. Vet. Med Assoc. 171, 171–177.

Williams, J.T., Dick Jr., E.J., VandeBerg, J.L., Hubbard, G.B., 2009. Natural Chagas disease in four baboons. J. Med. Primatol. 38, 107–113.

Wolf, A.F., 1969. Sensitivity to Triatoma bite. Ann. Allergy. 27, 271–273.

Wood, F.D., 1934a. Experimental studies on *Trypanosoma cruzi* in California. Proc. Soc. Exp. Biol. Med. 32, 61–62.

Wood, F.D., 1934b. Natural and experimental infection of *Triatoma protracta* Uhler and mammals in California with American human trypanosomiasis. Am. J. Trop. Med. 14, 497–517.

Wood, F.D., Wood, S.F., 1941. Present knowledge of the distribution of *Trypanosoma cruzi* in reservoir animals and vectors. Am. J. Trop. Med. 21, 335–345.

Wood, S.F., 1941a. Chagas disease (does it exist in men in Arizona?). Southwestern Med. April, 112–114.

Wood, S.F., 1941b. New localites for *Trypanosoma cruzi* Chagas in southwestern United States. Am. J. Hyg. 34, 1–13.

Wood, S.F., 1941c. Notes on the distribution and habits of reduviid vectors of Chagas' disease in the southwestern United States (Hemiptera: Reduviidae). Pan-Pacific Entomol. 17, 85–94.

Wood, S.F., 1941d. Notes on the distribution and habits of reduviid vectors of Chagas' disease in the southwestern United States (Hemiptera: Reduviidae). Pan-Pacific Entomol. 17, 115–118.

Wood, S.F., 1942a. Observations on vectors of Chagas' disease in the United States. I. California. Bull. South Calif. Acad. Sc. 41, 61–69.

Wood, S.F., 1942b. Reactions of man to the feeding of Reduviid bugs. J. Parasitol. 28, 43–49.

Wood, S.F., 1943. Observations on vectors of Chagas' disease in the United States. II. Arizona. Am. J. Trop. Med. 23, 315–320.

Wood, S.F., 1944a. Notes on the feeding of cone-nosed bugs (Hemiptera, Reduviidae). J. Parasitol. 30, 197–198.

Wood, S.F., 1944b. An additional California locality for *Trypanosoma cruzi* Chagas in the western cone-nose bug, *Triatoma protracta* (Uhler). J. Parasitol. 30, 199.

Wood, S.F., 1949. Additional observations on *Trypanosoma cruzi* Chagas, from Arizona in insects, rodents and experimentally infected animals. Am. J. Trop. Med. 29, 43–55.

Wood, S.F., 1950a. The distribution of California insect vectors harboring *Trypanosoma cruzi* Chagas. Bull. South Calif. Acad. Sci. 49, 98–100.

Wood, S.F., 1950b. Allergic sensitivity of the saliva of the western cone-nosed bug. Bull. South Calif. Acad. Sci. 49, 71–74.

Wood, S.F., 1951a. Bug annoyance in the Sierra Nevada foothills of California. Bull. South Calif. Acad. Sci. 50, 106–112.

Wood, S.F., 1951b. Importance of feeding and defecation times of insect vectors in transmission of Chagas' disease. J. Econ. Entomol. 44, 52–54.

Wood, S.F., 1952a. Mammal blood parasite records from southwestern United States and Mexico. J. Parasitol. 38, 85–86.

Wood, S.F., 1952b. *Trypanosoma cruzi* revealed in California mice by xenodiagnosis. Pan-Pacific Entomol. 28, 147–153.

Wood, S.F., 1953a. Conenose bug (Triatoma) annoyance and *Trypanosoma cruzi* in southwestern national monuments. Bull. South Calif. Acad. Sci. 52, 57–60.

Wood, S.F., 1953b. Conenose bug annoyance and *Trypanosoma cruzi* Chagas in Griffith Park, Los Angeles, California Bull. South Calif. Acad. Sci. 52, 105–109.

Wood, S.F., 1955. Conenose bug observations from 1954 from southwestern national monuments. Bull. South Calif. Acad. Sci. 54, 43–44.

Wood, S.F., 1956. Sylvatic *Trypanosoma cruzi* in Triatoma from southern Utah. Bull. South Calif. Acad. Sci. 55, 180.

Wood, S.F., 1957. Conenose bug *Trypanosoma* observations for 1955–56 from southwestern national monuments. Bull. South Calif. Acad. Sci. 56, 51.

Wood, S.F., 1958. Conenose bug and *Trypanosoma* observations for 1957 from southwestern national parks and monuments. Bull. South Calif. Acad. Sci. 57, 113–114.

Wood, S.F., 1959. Body weight and blood meal size in conenose bugs, Triatoma and Paratriatoma. Bull. South Calif. Acad. Sci. 58, 116.

Wood, S.F., 1960. A potential infectivity index for Triatoma harboring *Trypanosoma cruzi* Chagas. Exp. Parasitol. 10, 356–365.

Wood, S.F., 1962. Blood parasites of mammals of the Californian Sierra Nevada foothills, with special reference to *Trypanosoma cruzi* Chagas and *Hepatozoon leptosoma* sp. n. Bull. South Calif. Acad. Sci. 61, 161–176.

Wood, S.F., 1975. *Trypanosoma cruzi*: New foci of enzootic Chagas' disease in California. Exp. Parasitol. 38, 153–160.

Wood, S.F., Hughes, H.E., 1953. A mammal host of *Trypanosoma cruzi* Chagas in Griffith Park, Los Angeles, California Bull. South Calif. Acad. Sci. 52, 103–104.

Wood, S.F., Anderson, R.C., 1965. Conenose bugs (Triatoma) visit unoccupied boy's camp in Los Angeles. J. Med. Entomol. 1, 347–348.

Wood, S.F., Wood, F.D., 1961. Observations on vectors of Chagas disease in the United States. III. New México. Am. J. Trop. Med. Hyg. 10, 155–165.

Wood, S.F., Wood, F.D., 1964a. New locations for Chagas trypanosome in California. Bull. South Calif. Acad. Sci. 63, 104–111.

Wood, S.F., Wood, F.D., 1964b. Nocturnal aggregation and invasion of houses in southern California by insect vectors of Chagas disease. J. Econ. Entomol. 57, 775–776.

Wood, S.F., Wood, F.D., 1967. Ecological relationships of Triatoma p. protracta (Uhler) in Griffith Park, Los Angeles, California Pacific Ins. 9, 537–550.

Woods, J.P., Decker, L.S., Meinkoth, J., Steurer, F., 2000. Lymph node aspirate from a 4-month-old Mastiff with weight loss, lymphadenopathy, and pyrexia. Vet. Clin. Pathol. 29, 137–139.

Woody, N.C., Woody, H.B., 1955. (Chagas' disease). American trypanosomiasis. First indigenous case in the United States. J. Am. Med. Assoc. 159, 676–677.

Woody, N.C., Woody, H.B., 1961. American trypanosomiasis. I. Clinical and epidemiologic background of Chagas' disease in the United States. J. Pediatr. 58, 568–580.

Woody, N.C., De Dianous, N., Woody, H.B., 1961. American trypanosomiasis. II. Current serologic studies in Chagas' disease. J. Pediatr. 58, 738–745.

Woody, N.C., Woody, H.B., 1964. Chagas' disease in the United States of North America. Anais Congreso International sôbre Doença de Chagas. 5, 1699–1724.

Woody, N.C., Hernández, A., Suchow, B., 1965. American trypanosomiasis. III. The incidence of serologically diagnosed Chagas' disease among persons bitten by the insect vector. J. Pediatr. 66, 107–109.

Yabsley, M.J., Noblet, G.P., Pung, O.J., 2001. Comparison of serological methods and blood culture for detection of Trypanosoma cruzi infection in raccoons (Procyon lotor). J. Parasitol. 87, 1155–1159.

Yabsley, M.J., Noblet, G.P., 2002a. Seroprevalence of Trypanosoma cruzi in raccoons from South Carolina and Georgia. J. Wildl. Dis. 38, 75–83.

Yabsley, M.J., Noblet, G.P., 2002b. Biological and molecular characterization of a raccoon isolate of Trypanosoma cruzi from South Carolina. J. Parasitol. 88, 1273–1276.

Yadon, Z.E., Schmuñis, G.A., 2009. Congenital Chagas disease: Estimating the potential risk in the United States. Am. J. Trop. Med. Hyg. 81, 927–933.

Yaeger, R.G., 1959. Chagas' disease in the United States. Rev. Goiana Med. 5, 461–470.

Yaeger, R.G., 1961. The present status of Chagas' disease in the United States. Bull. Tulane. Med. Fac. 21, 9–13.

Yaeger, R.G., 1971. Transmission of Trypanosoma cruzi infection to opossums via the oral route. J. Parasitol. 57, 1375–1376.

Yaeger, R.G., 1988. The prevalence of Trypanosoma cruzi infection in armadillos collected at a site near New Orleans, Louisiana. Am. J. Trop. Med. Hyg. 38, 323–326.

Yaeger, R.G., D'Alessandro-Bacigalupo, A., 1960. Further studies on Trypanosoma cruzi in Louisiana. J. Parasitol. 46 (5, Sect. 2) Suppl., 7.

Yamagata, Y., Nakagawa, J., 2006. Control of Chagas disease. Adv. Parasitol. 61, 129–165.

Young, C., Losikoff, P., Chawia, A., Glasser, I., Forman, E., 2007. Transfusion-acquired Trypanosoma cruzi infection. Transfus. 47, 540–544.

Zayas, C.F., Perlino, C., Caliendo, A., Jackson, D., Martinez, E.J., Tso, P., Heffron, T.G., Logan, J.L., Herwaldt, B.L., Moore, A.C., Steurer, F.J., Bern, C., Maguire, J.H., 2002. Chagas disease after organ transplantation – United States, 2001. MMWR. Morb. Mortal. Wkly. Rep. 51, 210–211.

Zeledón, R., 1953. Manifestaciones alérgicas consecuentes a la picada de triatomas (Hemiptera: Reduviidae). Rev. Biol. Trop. 1, 17–20.

Zeledón, R., 1974. Epidemiology, modes of transmission and reservoir hosts of Chagas disease. In: Elliot, K., O'Connor, M., Wolstenholme, G.E.W. (Eds.), *Trypanosomiasis and Leishmaniasis with Special Reference to Chagas Disease*, Ciba Foundation Symposium 20 (New series), Elsevier Excerpta Medica, Amsterdam, pp. 51–85.

Zeledón, R., Rojas, J.C., Urbina, A., Cordero, M., Gamboa, S.H., Lorosa, E.S., Alfaro, S., 2008. Ecologial control of *Triatoma dimidiata* (Latreille, 1811): Five years after a Costa Rican pilot project. Mem. Inst. Osw. Cruz. 103, 619–621.

Zingales, B., Andrade, S.G., Briones, M.R.S., Campbell, D.A., Chiari, E., Fernandes, O., Guhl, F., Lages-Silva, E., Macedo, A.M., Machado, C.R., Miles, M.A., Romanha, A.J., Sturn, N.R., Tibayrenc, M., Schijman, A.G., 2009. A new consensus for *Trypanosoma cruzi* intraspecific nomenclature: Second revision meeting recommends TcI to TcVI. Mem. Inst. Osw. Cruz. 104, 1051–1054.

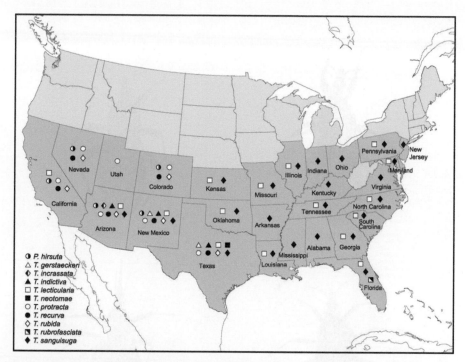

Plate 1 *Figure 2.1. Geographic distribution of U.S. triatomine species.*

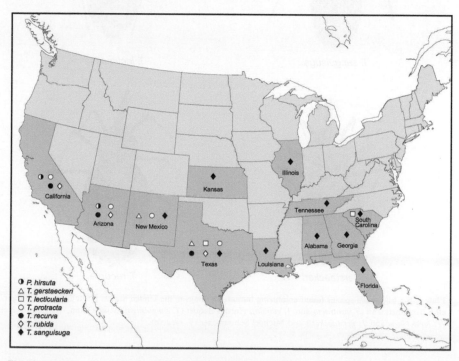

Plate 2 *Figure 2.2. Geographic distribution of species visiting households.*

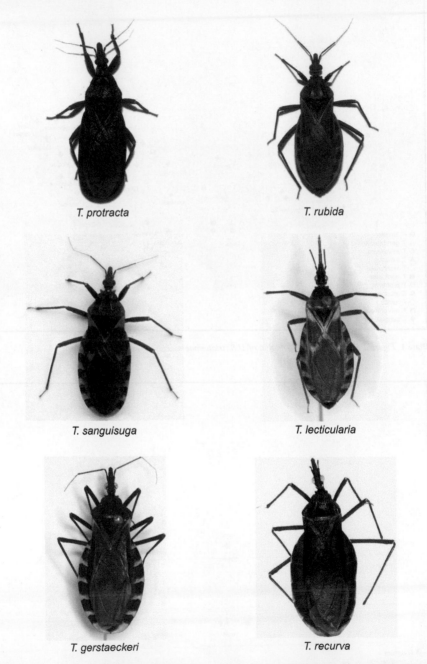

Plate 3 Six triatomine species found colonizing human dwellings in the United States. Photographers: Margarethe Brummermann (*T. protracta* and *T. rubida*), Harold Baquet (*T. sanguisuga*), Mike Quinn, TexasEnto. Net (*T. lecticularia* and *T. gerstaeckeri*) and Michael Schumacher (*T. recurva*).

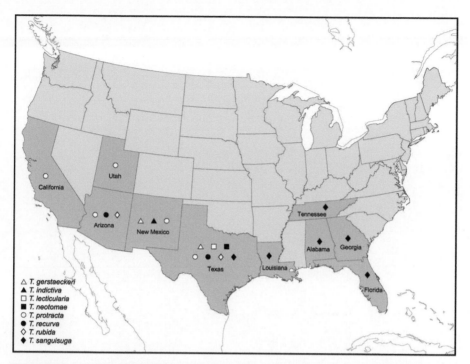

Plate 4 *Figure 2.3. Geographic distribution of species infected with* T. cruzi.

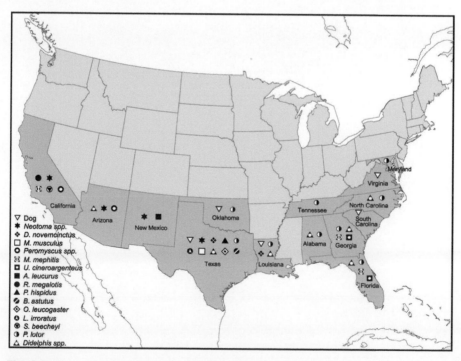

Plate 5 *Figure 3.1. Geographic distribution of known* T. cruzi *animal reserviors.*

Printed and bound by CPI Group (UK) Ltd, Croydon, CR0 4YY

03/10/2024

01040399-0012